P9-BJQ-203

All Thanks to God

# THE #1 HOW-TO COOKBOOK
# HOME COOKING
## TO
# CURE CANCER

## PREVENT, REDUCE, DESTROY, ELIMINATE, CURE

HEART ATTACKS,
ADD/ADHD, SIDS, COLDS, FLU,
DIABETES, WEIGHT, ALZHEIMERS,
ASTHMA, ARTHRITIS, ALLERGIES,
ACHES, PAINS, GLAUCOMA, AIDS &
ALL DISEASES!!

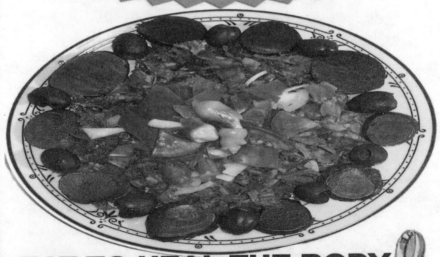

# EAT TO HEAL THE BODY
## RESTORE, REBUILD, REJUVENATE

Baby Miracle Survivor
The first & only
autobiography
cookbook
with a song!

# Jollie Harris III

This book is a survival story about a baby that became very sick, lost one of his senses, and was placed on a mission by God to share the light of how God can take a sad situation and turn it into a really great and wonderful thing, Called "the Miracle Boy" because he survived and beyond all beliefs, through God's food and the knowledge of the American Native Black Indians, he learned HOW TO become strong, healthy and whole again. NOW he helps you by revealing the secrets of HOW TO HEAL YOUR BODY naturally. See how to help yourself, and not rely on the help of others. You can cure yourself. Ü can cure Ü

## LET YOUR FOOD BE YOUR MEDICINE & YOUR MEDICINE BE YOUR FOOD

© 2004-2009 by Jollie Harris III

Feed God's Sheep Ministries All rights reserved.

All rights reserved. No parts of this publication may be recorded, reproduced, stored in a retrieval system or transmitted in any form or by any means electronic, mechanical, photocopying, or otherwise without the prior written permission of the copyright owner.

5TH EDITION          ISBN: 1-4116-1065-2
Published by UltimateLifeForce.com
Typesetting & composition by
                    HomeCookingCures.com

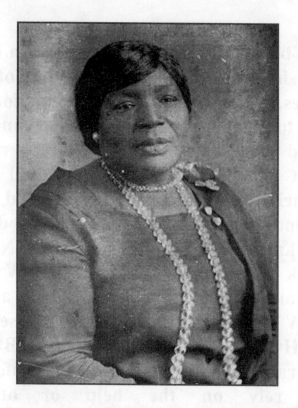

I'm thankful for my great grandma Alice Shivers; through her spirit I've acquired a lot of my cooking skills. I've also inherited her strong will to stand up for what I believe to be true. She was a Christian woman, powerful, and strong minded – the cook, nanny, and housekeeper for Augusta Busch, of Anheuser- Busch Beer of St. Louis, Mo. Her daughter was my grandma Bee who helped raise me.

I love her dearly.

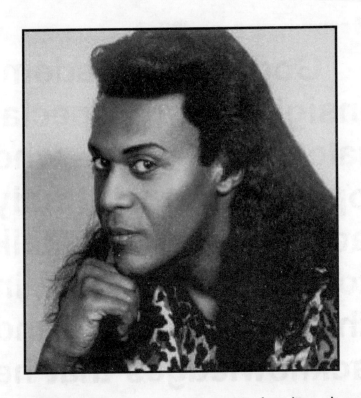

The author and servant who has been talking to God about spiritually healing the body for 45 years. Life has lead me to be a high profile personal assistant to many Royal families and also a personal assistant to homeless people in the street.

Now God has called on me to assist those with cancer. Believe me, in the area of personal assisting, I have paid my dues. Now God has called on me to assist you. I am your servant.

These blessings are from God and the Spirit of God's Foods.

**God gives wisdom, insight, and special talents to those who openly and faithfully accept the spirit, talk to the spirit, walk in the spirit and acknowledges that he or she is equal to and one with the spirit and all that God has made.**

**Jollie Harris III**
**Word of Wisdom**

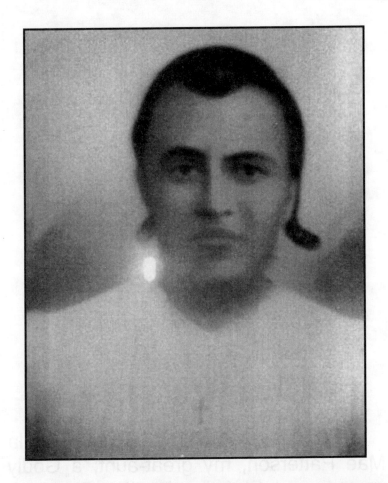

This is my great grandmother, LuNora Bratton, who is Cherokee Indian. She now lives in the spirit only. I love her very much. God has blessed me to talk to her Spirit for many years. My remedies are from her and my Indian Medicine Man great grandpa March McCallum.

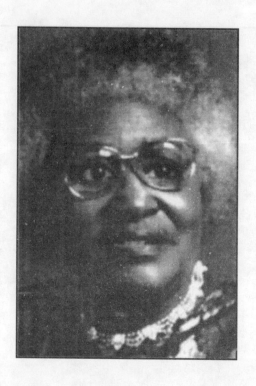

This book is also dedicated to Ella Mae Patterson, my great-aunt; a Godly woman and Christian Baptist. She took me to church as often as she could and helped me by giving all her heart to raise me and my sister Joyce while my parents went to work.

God bless Ella Mae Patterson and all of her 10 kids. I love you Ella Mae, with all my heart!

## Meet The Membership

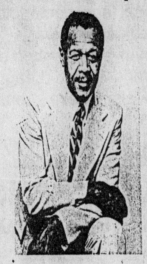

Jollie Harris is Chief of Building Management Service. As Chief, his responsibilities are directing a cleaning program designed to maintain the visual and bacteriological cleanliness of the Medical Center. The size and complexity of this facility has a direct impact on this service.

There are two divisions (Jefferson Barracks and John Cochran) approximately 17 miles apart. Cochran is in the inner city, high rise built in 1954; the other suburban spread out with multi-buildings (some built in 1922 and the rest in 1950).

The function of his position includes the following: herbicide/pesticide control, laundry/linen distribution, storing patients' effects, issuing indigent supplies, processing claims of patients loss or damage effects, mending, moving, furniture issue and storage, interior design, cleaning the environments, trash removal, signage program, odor control, light (candle power), etc.

His hobbies are video and tape recording and refurbishing houses.

He is currently involved in various organizations, such as Neighborhood Associations, Urban League, Synadical Task Force, Church Council, St. Louis Metropolitan Coalition, Member, St. Louis Association of Institutional Laundry Managers, Board Member and Program Chairman of National Executive Housekeepers Association, and a Member of the Educational Committee in the Missouri Hospital Association.

He has received a Superior Performance award, St. Louis Beautification award, North Parks Neighborhood award, Federal Women Program Certificate of Recognition, Certificate of Appreciation of Suggestion and Certificate of Merit for dedication during snowstorm.

This book is also in memory of my loving dad, whom I am very proud of. I wrote this book within two months of grieving over my dad, while the spirit was telling me that this was the way to keep my dad's spirit alive.

He was very educated and had 10-12 degrees in many subjects, and was an avid reader, leaving over 2000 books of every subject. He was a very active member in the Lutheran church and studied all religions.

He retired as the Chief of Building Management and Chief of Building Administration for the VA, - Veteran's Administration. His responsibilities were directing a cleaning program for the hospital and maintaining the visual and bacteriological cleanliness of the VA Medical Centers.

He was a very involved member of the Neighborhood Associations Urban League, a master gardener who also gave computer classes to senior citizens.

He was the block unit president and the host of the Jollie Harris Parade one day a year on Enright street in St. Louis MO where our home held the title and registration for being America's first block unit - block unit number one.

Most of the major city officials in St. Louis were present at his funeral.

This book is also dedicated to my mother, who loved my dad and stayed by his side. I love you Dorothy Harris.

She has volunteered many years to Habitat for Humanity and received many accomplishments and rewards, along with write-ups in local newspapers, and is today very healthy using my H.C.C.C. Program.

She has also spent time teaching an afterschool gardening program for kids.

# *Something to think about*

## ROAD 1.

Put your trust in God.
Love God and trust in God's
FOOD to HEAL the body
while loving yourself and
having the faith and
will to survive.

## OR

## ROAD 2.

Put your trust in doctor's, pills,
and the medical field.

Accept the stress, aggravation,
bills, loss of time and work –
now pray that there are no side
effects while wondering if the
pills ever worked or not.

*Which road will you take, 1 or 2?*

# The secret to curing cancer is knowing what foods to eat to stop the cancer, kill the cancer, and remove it safely from the body.

# Introduction
# GOD INSPIRED

This book is primarily written for those who are faced with a decision, but don't know where to go or what to do after a doctor has given you six months or less to live due to cancer, or any other blood and bacteria related diseases.

These doctors have run out of options; basically the doctor gives up because he or she has done all that they can, and their resources are limited and used up. They simply can't go any further.

Doctors have formats and prescriptions, where the Indian Medicine Men have wisdom, remedies and God's spirit.

This book is also a program which is spiritually designed to stop, reduce, and destroy cancer cells in your body by eating God's natural foods. This book does not follow any of man's rules, nor regulations for food and medical health. Nor does it follow textbook or literature formats. I am not a doctor - just a servant messenger.

This Home Cooking to Cure Cancer Program was formatted by God. Any person who follows this program will totally get the benefit of good health and happiness by preserving, rebuilding and extending life. My approach, spiritual instinct, grammar, and wording may not be something that you are familiar with. It may appear to be a bit offbeat to traditional book writing.

This book was not written for Mr. Critic, Mrs. Format or Mr. Grammar, nor is it written for a Pulitzer Prize or to be famous. It is written for those who are in need, love God, and are determined to beat cancer. In the spiritual healing world of wisdom, there is no such thing as grammar. Grammar is a man made thing. Therefore to master God's program you must in your mind and heart leave the world of man and enter the world of God.

The bottom line is that the foods I talk about in this book are all setting in your local produce departments. So you have    nothing to lose and so much to gain with a newly restored and healthy body. Most of you would not hesitate about restoring your face, hair, car, or your home.

Well, guess what - this is just a bit more important. Please read the philosophy of the book before you try the recipes. The knowledge of this simple program is the key to making the blessing work. I do not intend to offend anyone who does not believe in God. My belief is in Jesus Christ. So please read on and enjoy the blessing.

This book is in no way nor fashion to belittle or smear doctors, but to help draw you a picture so that you can see the difference between doctors, medicine, and their corporate commercials verses God, God's food, and your body.

Let us begin. On one hand we have people, whose greatest possession is their life and body. Most people, when they get sick, put their trust and life in the hands of doctors, medicine, and the Super Drugs we see on TV. Now let us flip the switch and put our trust in the hands of God, God's food - which was made to heal our bodies - and your own determination and will to get well.

These types of positive actions will certainly bring you Godly results and good health! Some of the reasons for so many deaths, diseases, cancer and so on are the pills, bad eating habits, overweight, lack of sleep, and the manufactured things we put in and on our body, be it food or other.

Right now let's paint you a picture regarding the pills. Here we are, living in a country with thousands of pills on the market - a billion dollar business. Most doctors, scientists, and I like to call the other guy's "laboratory cooks", who make up these pills with no proof that these pills are safe. They are new pills on the market. Oh well, the laboratory mice passed their test and now it is your turn.

Our doctors are not sure if these pills can be taken in conjunction with one another without causing great side effects. Nor do the doctors confer with one another while prescribing you these pills, which is one of the greatest mistakes in the medical industry. These doctors are guessing with your lives as to how these pills will react in your system and you are in the middle.

The same situation holds for in or out hospital patients. Some doctors give you experimental pills to take home for free, to see what the result will be. We as people should not have to live our lives as puppets to pill experiments - we deserve much more than to be cheated into paying millions of dollars for cold pills that don't work, and the medical industry confirms this while continuing to take your money.

Within the wisdom of this book you will find some words repeated. This is done on purpose with the intent of reaching your subconscious 2nd mind. This repetition allows your 1st mind to recall, understand, and see the clear visual picture of how you will heal your own mind, body and spirit.

Because of God's love and grace for you, the blessings of his food, has in the past and will forever in the future, allow you to be your own doctor of your own Holy Temple — Your Body!

The letter and text size in this book are intentional to help people with cancer that have problems staying awake, eating, reading and seeing.

**With each day I try to learn one thing, which makes that day, the Greatest Day Of My Life**

# HOME COOKING To CURE CANCER

# CONTENTS

# DRINK THE JUICE TO CURE

# THE BABY "MIRACLE BOY" SURVIVOR
## ABOUT THE AUTHOR

My name is Jollie Harris III. I was born in 1955 and raised in St. Louis Missouri.

Thank you for taking your time to hear a story about a little boy raised in a sterile room, and in a totally sterile environment.

My childhood and life began pretty much as a happy playful little boy, who was always running and hiding from bacteria. Dirt and just about any particles that flow through the air could make me sick.

Well, I'll tell you exactly how this began. I was about six months old and ate a very dangerous poison called Red Devil Lye. It was 100% pure. Lye in those days was known to be one of the deadliest poisons on earth - and it still is.

Lye is equivalent to liquid acid, but ten times stronger. It was used in many things such as Easy Bake Oven Cleaner, most brands of paint, Johnny on the Spots outdoor toilets; and the paint in the school playground equipment in the old days was based with Lye in the paint.

Nowadays, the school system has taken out all the old playground equipment and replaced it with new equipment that is not lye-based.

Grandma on the Beverly Hillbillies would always say to Jethro, "I'm going to wash your mouth out with lye soap." I think you Baby Boomers out there like me will remember that episode. Red Devil Lye if poured on concrete will burn a hole straight through, and you will see the smoke rising as it burns.

Just to give you an example of what the lye did to me when I was a baby - A mistake was made where my baby sitter and a family member were being distracted. Somehow I fell out of the bed and crawled into the room where the family member was cleaning the floor with Red Devil Lye, I knocked over the can, and licked the floor. This caused me to be rushed to the hospital to begin one of the most complicated surgeries in history and of my life.

The lye ate up and burned out my entire throat. My esophagus was gone-- finished-- the lye had burned straight through. The doctors had to rebuild and recreate my esophagus/throat in order for me to survive and stay alive.

I had a very good doctor. He told me later in life that I was the very beginning of his ear, nose, and throat career, which made him very successful. He said that God and God only pulled him through this operation. Thank You God for your Guidance of the hands of Dr. Gladny and Dr. Bond during this operation.

The lye that I ate just so happened to have a large picture of a Red Devil's face on the can. **I WILL NEVER FORGET IT!**

Dr. Gladny later told me that he had in the past only operated on frogs. He called me The Miracle Boy! I lived in a sterile room where I could never come out. Maybe for about 5½ years I lived there, total.

This is a place where some of the kids would get to go home on holidays or birthdays, but sad to say, I could not go and enjoy a day in life as other kids could. I was not expected to ever talk, do sports, to sing, dance, or anything else. I had many allergies at that time. I was allergic to just about everything and I had a very nervous stomach which was easy to upset. Anything that I ate would upset me in some kind of way. I could not swallow food.

My mother would come to the hospital everyday to visit me; she would put her hand on one side of the glass window to talk to me and I would put my hand on the other side of the glass - that's how we would talk to each other. I remember my feelings when I was four years old. It was cold in the sterile rooms; that's because bacteria feeds on heat and makes it grow faster. The glass I put my hand on felt cold to my heart knowing that I could not hug my mother on the other side of the glass.

There were many days I walked away from the glass with tears in my eyes because I could not go home with my mother. In this home, I had two strings coming out of each of my nostrils, tied to holes in the cartilage of my nose to keep the plastic tubes placed in my throat. These tubes were to force a reconstructed opening in my throat where Red Devil Lye Poison had burned and ate up my esophagus. I looked like a catfish with tubes in his throat, and that is just what the kids called me--Catfish.

The little girls would get their fingers tangled up in my strings and it would make me cry. I could feel the plastic tubes in my throat being yanked up and down as little girls accidentally got their hands and fingers caught in my strings. While playing I tried to have fun, but it was difficult.

My food was placed directly into my stomach by opening a piece of plastic and then sealing it tight to keep air and bacteria from getting in. The nurse would open the plastic, stick the food straight into my stomach, then the nurse would seal it tight and that's how I ate for many years with no food ever entering my mouth. The sense of taste was one of the five senses that I lost during those years. Sometimes air pockets would get into my stomach and made my stomach very nervous and upset. It felt like many heart attacks happening at the same time.

For the most part, all of my nurses were Catholic Nuns/Sisters, who worked at the Children's Hospital where I lived. These nuns and nurses wore long black robes with white hats that looked like they could fly. I called all the nuns in the hospital momma, maybe because I saw them every day. In my mind they were my mom, even though I did have a very good relationship with my mother whom I saw on a regular basis.

I really want to send special appreciation from my heart, to all the Nuns / Sisters / Nurses and Doctors that were there for me and helped me to recover. I also want to say thank you to the family members of those Nuns because they also share the same love and blood of these God Gifted people. Catholic Nuns / Sisters are God's chosen people. Nuns are some of the greatest people on the earth and still today have not achieved the respect, honor and recognition that they so rightfully deserve from the American public. America should celebrate the Nuns and make A Day for Nuns a national holiday.

We should never forget all of their countless hours of volunteer work - also helping and assisting the Red Cross for many years. I just want to say thank you God for sending your angels to earth, the

Nuns / Sisters! I love you all so much, may God keep on blessing you.

I would also like to acknowledge, say thanks, and pay a special respect to the Red Cross for the many years and days where your volunteers have lifted my spirit and heart doing their very best to assist me in any and every way possible. Mainly keeping me happy through the most difficult time of my life.

Now maybe all of you readers out there will understand why it is so important for me to be your servant. Life is a cycle of circles and I must give back to the universe. I pray that God will bless the Red Cross and everyone involved. My mother would come and see me every day.

In the hospital is where I started to learn about germs. Because I could not eat through my mouth or use my throat, I gained a very high keen sense of smell and sight.

I could smell and see bacteria in the air which might sound impossible. I would know when there was dangerous bacteria in my air space, simply by smelling it.

By six and seven years old I was able to talk fluently without pain. Thank God, finally, I could get out of the cold sterile room and could go home. Every year of my life after that till I was 21, I had to go back into the Hospital right when school was letting out for summer break and get operated on again. It took up my whole summer vacation. I remember trying to run away at the last day of school every year.

My parents would come to the school early on those days to put me back in the hospital. My dad was forced to grab me by my shirt collar as I tried to run away. I got very tired of having operations. All of my operations started off with a gas mask placed over my face as the doctors turned up the gas called ether. After my eighth or ninth surgery the gas/ether was not doing the job of sedating me or knocking me out as you would call it. So the doctors turned up the gas even more.

Many times I physically fought the doctors and nurses in the operating room. They taped me to wooden boards attached to the surgery bed and I looked like Frankenstein with needles poked into my skin everywhere they could put them, trying to sedate me.

Twice I woke up in the middle of surgery and I responded like a gorilla. It was a horrible scene. Looking at all the scalpels and knives made me hysterical. A patient must be totally relaxed before they go under in a surgery room or it can cause many complications. This is why many people die during surgery due to complicated situations and the family never knows because they cannot see what is going on in a surgery room.

I deeply feel that laws should be changed where a family member who wants to view their love one in surgery room has the option to do so. By doing this, doctors and surgeons would be forced to take better precautions. Taking this action would lower the fatalities of malpractice deaths due to complicated surgeries.

Back at home it took a while for my brain to clear up from the ether. Sometimes it would take about a month or two for the ether to totally clear my brain. It was a groggy feeling as if you had sniffed the largest bag of glue on the planet or taken an overdose of PCP.

I would tell my father and friends after my brain had totally cleared up that I could see molecules and atoms in the air, but no one would ever believe me. They thought that it was impossible. I could see things in the air that looked like floating molecules everywhere I went. They were clear in the air and slowly floating by. Very tiny specks of different shapes but they were outlined and very visual to me. These molecules and atoms were visually clear to me up until the age of 30.

At ten years of age God let me know that I had a special gift, and that God had saved me for a special reason, to talk to people about poisons in my body, the bacteria, side effects, and to reverse side effects of my life.

Most of my dreams from ten to forty years of age were of me flying physically in the air. At this early age of ten, I did not see how anyone would listen to me. I could smell and sense germs and bacteria on someone's body, a blowing sent of bacteria in the air or on a person's breath, which would seriously irritate me. I also had to stand on the concrete pavement whenever I went to the park because I was allergic to the smell of grass, cut or uncut. The smell of it would ruin my day.

There are many types of bacteria so get ready for it, because as long as we are alive bacteria will be fighting to attack us. New bacteria pop up every day. There could be volumes of books filled with only the names of all the various types of bacteria. Many forms of bacteria, doctors and scientists will never know about, because it cannot be picked up by microscopes, lazar body scanners, biopsies, nor in the blood.

Our problems are with bad bacteria. The bad ones outweigh the good ones. A good bacteria for example is the bacteria in molded bread. My dad would take molded bread and make cookies and bake a cake with it. Early American Black Indians such as my great grandpa used bacteria formed mold as the original Penicillin.

For some reason at an early age, I was interested in why doctors do what they do. Now that I was getting a little older my doctors were prescribing me 10 mg valium pills at about the age of 12 years old.

These pills were given to me because I had an over active thyroid problem - the same problem that a lot of children have today with moving too fast, which gets them into trouble. This causes children physical problems by injuring their own bodies due to not paying attention and moving too fast. I knew what these pills were; they would get me high and slow me down. I wanted to slow down, but not that way, and guess what - I never took those pills. When the coast was clear, I threw my prescription pills away!

My dad was a male nurse at one time and had a den / library in our home with most of the top medical books you could find. I would study the doctors P. D. R's. I knew all about the pills, what they did, what they were made of, and all the companies they were made by. I also knew the manufacturers who were new on the market - up and coming - and I knew whether their pills were new experimental drugs being marketed for the first time, or pills from companies with a more proven track record of reliability and performance of their pills. And which pills were sold while still under the microscope with mice, testing, and investigating their side affects at the same time these unproven and skeptical pills are sold to you.

I remember telling my friend at 12 years old, if your mother keeps taking those pills, they are going to mess her up. Well, a few weeks later, his mother had a stroke; it made me feel very sad because I loved his mother very much, and I had seen and read the twelve pill bottles by her bed side and I knew this would happen. My insight about health and medicine at an early age was something that most people would never experience in life and never understand.

In the health medical world, I believe that God gave me a natural, extra sensory perception, just as he would do for the animals in the wild. God gives them their own individual instinct and perception to keep them healthy and safe. Some animals he gave extra sight, extra smell, or hearing.

It is very possible that God gave me this insight to protect my health due to losing my sense of taste and to help me rebuild my immune system through a life of living with severe poisoning, while at the same time knowing the love that I have for him.

Within this love and relationship that I have for God and the Sprit, God has taught me how to eat and cook to heal my body. This has been going on ever since I was 10 years old and in the Boy Scouts. My mother had a garden where she grew just about anything and everything you could think of. Growing gardens at home secures your family's health. So I began to pick a fruit or vegetable and to center my mind on it and learn how it worked and applied to my body.

I first began with the mustard green and the watermelon. My grandfather gave me the idea of the mustard greens which were growing in my mother's back yard. The watermelon was chosen because it is the number one fruit that everyone ate in my home town of St. Louis, Missouri.

I went crazy on eating these two foods for a period of three years under observation and learned how they heal the body. The watermelon is good to eat all the way down to the hull. The watermelon was a complete brain stimulator, a great energy boost; it rejuvenates the skin and helps your blood flow.

If you eat an enormous amount it will flush your kidneys, bladder, pancreas, and help promote stronger bones. I know because I ate watermelons for three days without my mother knowing it.

The watermelon is an exceptional fruit. The redder and sweeter watermelon promotes a stronger and longer life. As to the mustard green you will find quite a bit of information on it in this book. But I will tell you for now that the mustard green and the watermelon did a great big help and service to me with a problem I had with some reverse affects from my surgeries.

I use to jump in a jolting, jerky motion. It caused me at one time in school to drop my lunch tray on another kid at school and it was very embarrassing. As I grew older it would affect me when I drove my car. I would get little jolts between 3 and 10 times a day. It was a very painful and a strange pain to the right or to the left body motion. I also had another problem where it felt like someone laced a long string with tiny small pieces of glass glued onto a string, then began to pull it, starting between my legs and ripped up through my stomach and chest. This heart ripping painful motion went on for many years.

When I started eating the mustard green and the watermelon I noticed the painful number of incidents slowed down. I was thanking God that these two items - when I ate them on the same day - solved my symptoms, and they kept on working in amazing ways.

The doctors use to tell my mother that the pain was all in my head, that I was lying, and they prescribed water pills to fake me out. I told the doctor wait till I tell my dad. The doctor would tell me, "I'm still going to bill your mom and dad"!

Prescribing water pills to people has been a silent financial gravy train to doctors for many years. People take these pills for many years and never say anything to the doctors about the pills not working and doctors are aware of this. People think that they can't speak against a doctor. They think that they are putting the doctor down or verbally shaming the doctor, if they were to speak up. By all means they should.

On the other hand, because my situation was so severe, I would not allow any intern doctors to start a conversation with me. Interns are what I call practicing doctors fresh out of school. I would always say go away and find another guinea pig. They always wanted to come over to me look down my throat and press on my stomach. I knew that my illness was very rare and many doctors from around the world wanted to meet me, but this was getting to be a bit ridiculous.

Sometimes I was a little rude with those doctors. I thought they would mess me up as soon as they got me on the operating table because I wouldn't let them press on my stomach and I gave them a hard time. As a kid I had to do what I had to do and say what I had to say. After thousands of doctors and interns pushing on me I felt like a pin cushion. My parents could not help me when I was one on one with a doctor or in an operating room.

I said all this to say, "Hold on, if there is no hope in sight, you can always lean on God." Remember, it is always darkest before the dawn and where there is God, there is a Way!

God is good all the time. You just have to have faith and look deep into the spirit and you will always find God's goodness. Now today God has taken a young boy who was raised in a sterile room with a reconstructed throat/ esophagus. A boy who could not eat through his mouth without pain for about 16 years, and who the doctors said would never be able to talk, nor perform any athletic activities, nor play as other kids do.

Well, people, I am standing here to say that God has blessed me with the gift of life, singing like a bird and playing the guitar. This has been my work for the past 33 years as a Singer/Performer. Singing from St. Louis, Missouri to Royal Families, in small Bistro Cafés and numerous West Hollywood and Beverly Hills 3, 4, and 5-star restaurants, night clubs, several country clubs, and some very posh places in and out of the country.

God has also blessed me with the ability to run track for four years in high school and win first place in the state competition each year and do karate as a sport. God has blessed me with beautiful family members and a child. God has blessed me to be a personal assistant to Royal Families, Super Stars and Homeless People in the street.

Now God has blessed me for the past 35 years with the art of helping people with their health and weight problems, fighting colds, cancer, kidney, and memory disorders, and so on. This is something that I have always done of free heart and spirit, good will to woman- and man-kind.

Never ever, I repeat never ever has money been involved. And never ever was, nor is, any type of pharmaceutical medicine involved. I simply hate medicine and I refuse to be a "Puppet to Pills", including any type of vitamins in any pill form, nor cold medications.

Pills in most cases are psychological training wheels, which need to come off. I only deal with God's food, good conversation and talking to you about what foods to eat, how to cook them, and how they heal and relate to the body.

My talent and knowledge of God's food is extremely rare and my food program is unknown to man and woman kind. But trust me; all of God's animals instinctively understand my program, simply because my program is their program. And believe that their program is not the program of mice and rats that are tested in laboratory experiments.

These so called conclusions have led to the invention of millions of pills, that have failed the American public over the last 50 years and which have destroyed and killed millions of lives. Remember at one time doctors didn't believe that washing their hands was totally necessary before, during, and after surgery. During that time people were dying like flies. Doctors at that time needed to be corrected and updated.

The same updates and corrections are needed today with the doctor's old fashioned laboratory mice experiments. Mice have a total different system than humans. Along with roaches, they have the most complicated systems to kill and destroy, so how do we compare?

I have never in my life seen a human enter a house by making their bodies flat like a rat and sliding under a door, nor by coming into your house by way of the toilet. Today, doctors and scientists still need to be reformed and God is the only reform school!

Somehow the medical industry does not want to change for the better. They insist on playing marketing mind games with the help of large corporations and insurance companies. Maybe it's all about money and population control. One thing for sure is, it's not about God.

The reason I have so much to say is that I fear no man, only God and God only. Many people whom I have helped feel that God has truly shown me the vision of his food in a talented way that can easily be expressed to others. God's food is a total miracle and the world's best known secret, that needs to be told.

Many of my friends also call me their Guardian Angel who looks over their health. God's spirit as a servant has always led the way for me. My dad Jollie Harris Jr., who has recently passed on into the spirit, has also given me a vision to write this book to compile everything that he has taught me.

Now I dedicate this book to you, the reader. My theory is that of my Cherokee ancestry, and God's theory on food, where we believe that God's food should correspond together with the mind body and spirit.

Some of the items that I talk about come from the Bible, such as mustard leaf, mustard seed and mustard greens. If you'd like to read it yourself, you can read it in your Bible - "Mark chapter 4, verse 30-32:" Other good sources are bee pollen and pomegranate juice - they are favorite topics of mine.

Bee pollen is the world's most totally balanced and complete food of the universe. Bee pollen, bee honey, royal jelly are all product of the bees, which in history were mixed in the bread called manna eaten by the wise men on their journey through the desert.

So here it is clear and simple - if we only eat the foods that come out of the ground that God has created for us to eat, we would not be having problems of death due to diseases, nor this conversation.

Each country in the world has been set up by God with different foods, fruits, olives, vegetables, and grains. When the people in each of these countries, around the world, get involved and seek to find the foods that best work for them. Each food has a different relationship with your body's health. Foods that grow from the ground. Some foods, when combined together, solve specific problems in the body. I buy most of my food from the local produce departments at the local store, and from international food stores. These stores are where you generally find people from the Middle East shopping.

People from the Middle East and Far East countries, for thousands of years, have been eating good foods that benefit their body's health and wellbeing, such as Japan, China, Korea, and the Philippines, Africa, Saudi Arabia, Lebanon, Syria, Spain, Italy, Greece, Africa, Jamaica and

India. God naturally grows the foods for these people in their countries, and he does the same for us here in America.

Basically I will be your guide to which foods do what and how they apply to healing the body. Also, I will be showing you how to cook to stop the spread of cancer, to rebuild your immune system, fight bacteria, replenish your blood cells with oxygen, lower blood pressure, cut and reduce cholesterol levels, also lower your sugar and salt intake while losing weight, all in one meal.

You may say to yourself that it is impossible for a meal to save a life. God has many wonders, and I thank him for the blessings of allowing me to be your servant and good-spirited messenger of God's foods and the wonders of how they heal. God's not going to give up on you. You only have to make one step, as he makes two.

My grandmother would always say, I may give out but I will never give up, so give yourself another chance!

# THE COMMON COLD & FLU CURE

*They say there is not a cure for the common cold but this is not true. Here is my formula through the spirit of God.*

1. Babies with colds - feed fresh crushed apples; mix in 1/3 banana. Crush in a form that is very soft and digestible, like apple sauce that you made yourself. Do the same with the banana. A natural way is to wash your finger tip very clean and put one drop of raw honey on your finger tip. Add the apple mixed with banana and feed it to your baby - your baby will love it. Your baby will feel the love through your fingers and mentally feel comforted at the same time. Do this in the morning and at noon but not before bed time at night.

2. Children - feed them 3 apples a day and a small mustard green salad. Add whatever your child likes to the salad – tomatoes, mushrooms,

whatever. Spray this salad 5 times with brown APPLE CIDER VINEGAR (the brown) and 8 times GRAPE SEED OIL. Squeeze lemon juice over the top and maybe add a little of your child's favorite cheese over the top.

3. Adults - eat all the above plus a large mustard green salad. Add olives, curry, squeezed lemon juice, tomatoes, beets, radishes, spray heavy with brown APPLE CIDER VINEGAR (the brown only) and extra virgin olive oil or GRAPE SEED OIL. Spray double the amount of oil as you do the vinegar.

Adults with the flu - put 2 shots of golden apple cider vinegar, 2 crushed garlic, 2 spoons of raw honey into a 4-ounce glass of tea that you made with the mustard green curly leaf, and drink it.

You can also drink 100% grape juice - it has ten times the vitamin C as an orange - and get plenty of rest. The grape juice will turn your bowels the color black but it's ok; it will clear in 3 days.

Our choices of healing are a lot better if we allow God, who is the master and the creator of our body, to take charge, and to respect the food he placed in the ground to heal and nourish our body. Remember you are what you eat.

There are a lot of good doctors out there and a lot of bad ones. When I was 12-18 years of age you could hold up a pill in the air and I could tell you what it was and how it would affect your body, and sometimes exactly how many milligrams.

I read the Doctors P.D.R.s every day. My dad use to test me on them for punishment. Whenever I did something wrong he made me read medical books for days on end and questioned me later. I knew more than most doctors about pills at an early age.

Because of my eating poison and living in the hospital for 5 years, and after about 21 operations, I have learned the in and outs of hospitals, medical clinics, surgery rooms, all forms of medicines, the pharmaceutical industry, also the trickery of puppet pill marketing, good and bad doctors and who's playing the game on who.

My dad also retired as the Chief of Building Management and Administration for America's Veterans Hospitals. Anything that I did not know regarding the medical industry, my dad has taught me the rest. God bless my dad Jollie Harris Jr. in Heaven. I love you always.

My dad always wanted me to be a doctor because he felt that I had it in me.

I always wanted to be a Singer /Musician and a Food Medicine Healer and that's what I am. I never liked the pharmaceutical part of health, after knowing so much about it, nor did I ever in my life like taking pills.

# THE POWER OF GOD'S FOOD

The power of God's food is one of God's most important blessings, which cures, feeds, and nourishes the body. Humans overlook, do not understand, do not have time for, and will live out their entire life missing the blessings of God's food and how it applies to us and our bodies. People worldwide and the average American person would rather rely upon the doctors, pills, commercials marketing, and other advertisement agencies which are sponsored by large corporations, to control their health, their life, and their money.

It's about time we as people wake up and realize that we should be putting our health, our life, and our money in the hands of God instead of man. Up until now you simply have been paying doctors, corporations, and insurance companies for your BAD HEALTH. I repeat BAD HEALTH. Some doctors and corporations are good and tell you the truth about your health, food, body and nourishment, but most don't. It is up to us as God's children, whose bodies are designed, operated, crafted, controlled, and spirited by GOD to remember to keep the faith, and that God is the giver of birth and the taker of life on this planet.

## It's All About God
## Hopefully you get the point!

# A TRUE TESTIMONY OF JOLLIE HARRIS III

There is no man on this earth who can take this knowledge away from me. Very few people in America have experienced my type of illness and lost their sense of taste (because I could not eat through my mouth and have lived for so long in a sterile room free of bacteria).

God has saved my life from the Red Devil Lye Poison I ate as a baby. God has also called upon me to tell the world how God has given me the insight to heal my own body through the Power of God's Foods.

My stomach was one of the most sensitive and most nervous stomachs on the planet. Any level of bacteria from anywhere would make me sick, and was critical to my condition in those days. I was also raised with an over active thyroid, what some people now call Attention Deficit Disorder.

This information is now due to the American public because the malpractice of the medical industry is killing too many of God's people! God will bless all these people in Heaven who died trying to fight for their lives while going through years of being ripped off by Medical Malpractice. Malpractice needs to be called out on the carpet so that it can be accounted for the dead in which it truly does, which is a high rate of killing thousands of people.

Too many people are dying and having complications due to pills, doctor neglect and simple surgical mistakes. Doctors and nurses are overworked for too many hours and have too many patients on the schedule to give proper care and attention to any one patient. There should be a law to regulate the amount of surgeries a doctor can perform in a day based upon the intensity of the surgery, the stress of the surgery, and the actual time it takes to do the surgery.

Also nurses should work fewer hours to prevent mistakes. Patients and patient's families should be well aware if there is a switch hitter or substitute surgeon acting in place of the originally agreed surgeon.

The patient should be able to talk to that surgeon if the patient can talk. This gives security to the patient's mind in knowing who is going to do the surgery.

I had a surgery go bad once in my teens because I did not like the new switch hitter surgeon who was assigned to me. As a result I had a bad recovery and needed to go back and get the surgery done over. Right before a person goes under they know for sure if they trust or like the surgeon.

The anesthesiologist is another person that the patient must get along with or feel trust in. Over-sedating a patient for many years has also been another major malpractice problem which causes many severe complications.

You have the right, as a patient, to feel secure because it's your life, and you or your family member had to sign on the dotted line and you pay and agree to the acknowledgement that any complications during surgery could be fatal. That is how the hospital and surgeons are not responsible for their malpractice neglect!

Families should have a long, in-depth conversation regarding all in- and out-patient surgeries. To everyone who has died due to malpractice neglect, I dedicate from my heart this book to you. Many of you were cancer patients.

**CHILDRENS HOSPITAL** WAS WHERE I LIVED IN **ST. LOUIS** AS A BABY. IT IS ALSO WHERE I HAD ALL OF MY OPERATIONS DUE TO THE **RED DEVIL LYE POISON**. JUST TO SHOW YOU THE POWER OF GOD, THE PLACE WHERE THE **ANGELIC NUNS** WORKED, AND THE HOSPITAL I WAS IN IS ON **"KING'S HIGHWAY"**.

# NOT ALL DOCTORS ARE BAD

Please do not misunderstand me by thinking that I am saying all doctors are bad. For example, my child's doctor is excellent and he wins many awards because of the way he cares for his patients. There are many good doctors out there who really care about their patients and love God before money. These doctors are heaven-sent and extremely hard to find. So when you find a good doctor never let him go!

**GOD BLESS THE GOOD DOCTORS AND THEIR GOOD WILL**

Over 200 years ago the Native Indians and Black Indians were trying to teach early American settlers the value in eating properly. During this time, men and women's food sources were primarily animals - meat which was killed in the woods. Soon these settlers got tired of the meat and needed more nutrients to survive. The Indians taught them how to grow different crops and cultivate the land.

God's food is the only natural cancer cure! Man has caused his own destruction with the invention of new foods, food processing additives, preservatives, the adding of sugar, salt and pasteurization, toxins in the air and house hold cleaning supplies. Each and all of these ingredients make up new forms of bacteria, which we today call cancer. This is what most of us are living with from day to day.

This also explains why so many new people are getting cancer today. Two hundred years ago we did not have all these products on the market - now we do.

People with cancer should take golden brown APPLE CIDER VINEGAR baths with one quart of golden brown APPLE CIDER VINEGAR in their bath tub water to clear skin of toxins and bacteria. Do not wash clothes in bleach - use one cup of golden apple cider vinegar in the washing machine.

Cancer also comes in the form of stress and, believes me; the stress of dieting also causes thousands of people cancer, which will grow at a slow rate over a period of years. I am 100% against the word *diet* - it is a very dirty four letter word in my vocabulary, which the American public has become accustomed to.

This crazy marketing technique is a growing and thriving billion dollar business. Stressful dieting can cause the brain to release fluids in your body which breeds very dangerous bacteria and causes you cancer. Forget the word diet and learn my system of eating the proper foods from your local produce department and the Almighty God will take you the rest of the way. You make one big step and God will make two.

All this information that God has revealed to me is so much clearer than the water you drink.

To relieve stress from cancer patients, a good idea is to watch a lot of movies, especially funny movies. Or maybe go out and play bingo, do something that's a little physical like walking. Try to do something that makes you happy and makes the time go by without you having to think about it.

Whatever stresses you out; it is your job to push it aside, including your bills. Learn how to look at your bills when you are in a good mood or during one of your happier moments.

# THE CANCER CURE WALK

Let's talk about walking for just a moment. "God made the Heart to Automatically Tune Itself". All you have to do is walk properly. I'll show you how.

When you walk, swing your arms - try to swing your arms high and parallel to your shoulders. When you step your left leg out, raise your right arm parallel to your shoulder. When you step your right leg out, raise your left arm up, parallel and even to your shoulder. Walk until you get sweat on the top of your head, at this point your heart is pumping at God's ratio and tempo.

This is God's program for a naturally tuned heart. Walking this way will lower your blood pressure, reduce cancer, reduce your sugar, reduce weight, help you to digest your food, help you to get a good night's sleep, help you to dream, trim your body fat, and give you a better overall appearance.

This is just one of God's greatest blessings, so tune up your heart - it's natural and free! There is no pill or doctor that can possibly do for you what you can do for your heart by simply walking the proper way. Ancient monkeys standing upright would swing their arms while walking. Many armies around the world marched this way to give strength to their men in battle - the American army does not, nor do any of our armed forces.

To take your walking a step further and turn it into a total power walk, breathe in when you step out with your left leg and your right arm up. Breathe out when you step out with your right leg and your left arm up. The trick is to keep your arms parallel even to your shoulder, not higher not lower.

The constant penetration of air to the upper respiratory system and lungs on a regular basis help respiratory problems and asthma patients. Example: If you were an alcoholic or chain smoker, the perpetual moving of doing the proper walk twice a day, morning and night, helps you to slowly reduce your cravings of smoking and drinking, by sending a signal to your brain that your chest wants to breathe air freely.

# ANOTHER
# WORD
## OF
# WISDOM

God has blessed a woman's body to bear children. The first years for men and women on earth were about a chain of command. Respecting God, respecting the woman from which children are born. Respecting God's food which he placed on earth for our nourishment, health, mental capacity and survival. Also respecting the land, sea, ocean, sky and God's animals.

Men through history and today's men who rule the world do not respect God, women, God's food, and God's kingdom. Men do not respect women as to God's expectations of how God feels a man should respect a woman, and so it is that man has broken all links of the chain of command which guides him to good health and survival. Man has now caused his own self destruction.

The moral of this story is, respect God, respect women and children, then respect God's almighty good food and environment. If man and woman could follow the chain of command, men and women's food could digest properly in a Godly way, giving you a better night's sleep, therefore allowing the body to heal itself, giving you what we all want, which is better health and long happy life.

A world without the insight and guidance of a woman is a life half-lived. My life must be full and complete and not a half. Therefore I am a God fearing man who loves and respects women, children, old people, God's food, his animals, and environment, which all adds up to making me a Happy Healthy Stress Free Guy, allowing my food to bring me maximum nourishment to heal my body - and so can you. Just follow these steps and stay with the spirit of God.

# CANCER AND WOMEN

Hello women, God wants me to express to you with all my heart that cancer is greatly caused by what we put on the exterior of our body and on the inside. It is also due to long-term toxic buildup in and on our body and brain, which all has to go somewhere, and guess where it goes? It becomes Bacteria/Cancer.

Ladies, I pray that each and every one of you would hear my cry as to your concerns regarding cancer.

In America today, 2 out of every 4 women will get some form of cancer. The reason why so many women today are multiplying in numbers with cancer is that in the 50s, 60s, and the 70s we had fewer items and products on the market which are made for women. But in today's world there are millions of products for a woman to buy and apply to her body and in her body.

Just about everything that is marketed to women today can ultimately give her cancer. These products are marketed and sold, and millions of these products are not properly tested. These companies and corporations continue to put these products on the market and we still today don't know if they have any long term effects, or long term adverse effects. This epidemic is becoming very dangerous to women and I have known this for about 35 years.

Here is a small list of items which give women cancer:

Hair sprays,
Lotions,
Face makeup,
Fabric coloring in underwear,
Thongs make vaginal infections,
Shaving items,
Lipstick,
Eye makeup,
Tanning supplies and tanning booths,
Finger nail polish and polish remover,
Wrinkle removers,
Facial creams and facial mask,
Slim down weight candy bars,
Energy drinks,
Too much sun,
Diet pills,
vitamin pills,
Food supplement pills,
Home cleaning supplies.

The water you drink--it's all bad. Use distilled or mineral water instead.

Your shower water has chlorine/bleach in it. Use filtered shower heads.

Body building foods, drinks, candy bars, diet foods and their supplements grow cancer.

Now there is a new one on the market that claims to be a spray on stocking. I wonder what type of toxins and chemicals it brings and who paid for their safety inspections.

I feel that women should stand up, hear my cry, and see with open eyes that there is an open market rush of dangerous and harmful products sold to women everyday in America and in a very global way!

A good rule of thought is, when a new product is introduced on the market, take a moment to think in your mind, "Does this product appear to have natural ingredients from the ground or is it totally chemically manufactured?"

If you feel that it is chemically processed and manufactured then there is a strong possibility of this item giving you cancer. Women, I know that you are listening. Please use as many items or products that you can which are natural or as close to natural as possible. This is the key to preventing the risk of cancer.

Let's keep it simple and keep it in mind that there are some companies out there who market natural products which are a good thing for women. Hopefully the natural product market will in the near future overpower and knock out the chemical beauty products, and secure their safety - a new day for women!

Also remember everywhere you get the most sweat, your head, armpits, vaginal area, your anal area and between your toes may cause cancer. So keep your body clean and use the bath tub to help prevent these problems. For example: a loofah to wash and clean your face with is all-natural; it grows from the ground.

The loofah restores and vitalizes the skin while removing layers of dead skin cells, which we must do to have vibrant and healthy skin. The loofah also cleans your pores, gets rid of pits, zits, other toxins and pollution, and it's cheap to buy. This will allow you that beautiful glow.

Using 100% Cocoa Butter is a perfectly healthy moisturizer for your face. It comes in a stick - the brand I use is Woolies 100% stick Coco butter. It is also great for that even tone and the perfect tan, allowing your skin to glow. It gives elasticity and life back to your face. By the way, the answer is no, I do not work for any product or food suppliers!

**In the arena of cancer, women get hit the hardest and get the shorter end of the stick. There needs to be a change in these surging high numbers. The average number of girls born in America is much greater than boys, so girls, young females and the women of America are at a much higher risk than they think!**

Remember - it's your life and stress is your enemy; it helps cancer grow. Reducing your weight, and your salt and sugar intake, can also reduce stress. Try not getting upset or mad - this places tension on your muscles, releasing a fluid which is stress related, causing you a faster cancer growth. Stress is a very tricky thing which breaks down the body in every area and comes in many forms of life.

# THE BIG C
# AND
# 10 DAYS LEFT TO LIVE

A true story about meeting Mrs. X, a terminally ill Latino princess from Guadalajara, Mexico, while at the same time being lifted by God to help this person, giving me the insight and wisdom while placing my faith in God's food to help, heal and destroy cancer.

I call her a princess because this lady has a heart of gold. It's quite interesting how we met.

I was singing one night in a local Beverly Hills restaurant. On my break that night I met a woman who told me that she loved my singing. I said "thank you very much" and asked the lady to come back and see me the following week. She said "I can't" and I said "Why not?"

Then she dropped her head and said, "I can't because I'm going to die before next week." Mrs. X weighed about 85 pounds soaking wet, five feet four inches tall, and very weak, she could hardly stand up on her feet. She could not stay awake over three to four hours, could not keep her food down, had not properly used the restroom in several months. She told me that her doctor had given her 10 days to live. At the time I met her she had about 5 days left. He also told her that she was fully blown with cancer from head to toe.

The doctor prescribed Prozac for her depression and told Mrs. X that her cancer stages were too far advanced and that chemo/radiation would not help her. The doctor told Mrs. X to go home, take the Prozac, and die peacefully.

Hearing this knocked me clear off my feet. Finally I realized that Mrs. X was out trying to enjoy what she thought were her last days. Then a light came on in my head that God had healed my body by food, and that this was the right time to be a servant and messenger to Mrs. X.

I had always had faith in God's power to heal the body through food. So I asked Mrs. X to let me help her, since all had failed as per her doctor. She had given up and had no hope. She replied, "I don't think that anyone can help me." I kept talking until I convinced her to allow me to help her.

I took her home and cooked for her for five days. She had problems eating, sleeping and going to the bathroom. The Prozac had her going and coming in and out of her mind. At times she did not know who she was. She would curse me out one day and apologize in sorrow and tears the next day. I knew it was the Prozac talking and taking over her brain, and she was considering suicide.

She had a very hard time keeping the food down; she would bring it back up. We kept on trying and I made her my Ultimate Mustard Green Tea.

## Ultimate Mustard Green Tea

Ultimate Mustard Green Tea with brown APPLE CIDER VINEGAR, garlic, lemon, honey, and slowly boiled mustard greens.

My recipe for this tea is, put ten tablespoons of brown APPLE CIDER VINEGAR in a cup with the squeezed juice of two lemons, three large spoons of honey, and three garlic cloves which you have crushed yourself by hand. Get three mustard green leaves and boil with distilled water in a small separate pot. Then strain mustard green tea and pour it into the cup with the brown APPLE CIDER VINEGAR, garlic, lemon, and honey.

This is my own creation for the ultimate tea that heals the body. It beats up on cancer, neutralizes the cancer, and feeds the immune system at the same time. Later we can flush the system through with 1/3 vinegar and 2/3 distilled water in a glass.

Due to vinegar being hard on the kidneys, drink plenty of water five minutes after consuming large amounts of brown APPLE CIDER VINEGAR (the brown only never the clear). Cancer patients should only use distilled water, or mineral water.

At times, drink water with two lemons squeezed in it. These type drinks will also heal the flu, colds  and infections in the body.

After three days she started keeping her food down and gaining about a half a pound a day. I could see her getting a bit stronger. I started to scream "Thank you God, Thank you God!"

I weighed her about three times a day. Kept track of the times she stayed awake. I also kept track of her bowel movements, making sure that they turned from black to brown, to light brown, to green, and that they floated on top of the water.

This might sound a little harsh to understand, but it is totally necessary in knowing how to treat the cancer problem, and that you have begun to cure the cancer problem. Also this lets you know that cancer has started to vacate the body.

Once again I am no doctor but God's Messenger and Servant Indian Spirited Food Healer, or what you may call a Modern Day Medicine Man, but remember I never use medicine.

Mrs. X could now stay awake through the day the more she ate God's food the less she felt the need to sleep or for Prozac. We took many walks. This was something she really did not want to do. She did not have much energy, but we walked further and further each day.

Cancer patients need someone by their side who they can trust, communicate with, and who understands their problem and has a positive attitude regarding the will to live.

We were on a major roller coaster ride with Mrs. X's brain because the Prozac had major side effects of mood swings and repeated suicidal tendencies. Thoughts kept running through my mind that the Prozac was making the cancer situation ten times harder to fight. Mrs. X's struggle was a fight for life.

At different times I would feed her, starting with large amounts of extra virgin olive oil to coat her stomach, and to get her stomach lining back in place, large amounts brown APPLE CIDER VINEGAR (the brown only). After the vinegar I would wait about 20 minutes to let the vinegar burn the cancer in God's natural way without using chemo, then flush her system down with about four large glasses of water.

I also fed her large amounts of mustard greens raw in a salad, cooked and juiced in a blender. I fed her these foods until she threw them back up - this was my way of knowing that her system had taken all the vitamins and minerals that God would allow her to take. I also gave her, 3 times a day, regular ¼ spoon amounts of raw, nonpasteurized bee pollen, 100% pomegranate juice, 100% grape juice, 100% cranberry juice, and lots of garlic, curry, tomatoes, beets, olives, radishes, and sometimes I would cook food with fresh habanera peppers in it.

By the way, the grape juice makes your bowels turn black but don't worry - it goes back to its natural color two days after you stop drinking it. It also loads your body with ten times the vitamin C as an orange and is equal to eating about one hundred carrot and celery sticks. This is my way of killing the cancer and rebuilding the immune system so that cancer does not come back, and of cleaning your colon at the same time. That's what this program is all about.

I would also feed her wild baked king salmon (not the farm grown) tomato soup (homemade), lentils and black beans with extra curry seasoning, a pinch of bee pollen, and Hummus with loads of garlic, and Tabouli salad. On the fifth day, she started to regain her faith in living and on this day she began to call me her Guardian Angel! She still calls me this today. I put a care package of food together for her.

Mrs. X and her ex-husband lived together - he came to pick her up from my home and said "thank you very much for the help". He was a super nice guy - a loving Christian man whom I respect very much. A few days later I drove to their home in Palm Springs and gave them my cooking recipes and instructions on how to cook the food, while her ex looked on.

He is a wonderful chef, and a great gourmet cook. This made everything easy. Thoughts of Mrs. X's teenage daughter kept running through her mind and gave her more inspiration to live. Today Mrs. X is living alive and well in Palm Springs, and is still a wonderful friend. This just goes to say,

## When All Fails, Keep the Faith and God Will Prevail!

# THE HOME COOKING TO CURE CANCER SECRET

Now is the time to tell you about my Greatest Secret, "Home Cooking To Cure Cancer". I believe that this is the answer the whole world has been waiting for, for so long.

It would not have been as great a help, or as great a service to you if I were to first show you my How To: Home Cooking to Cure Cancer Secrets and Recipes. This would not help you to clearly understand how to counter act stress which also causes cancer, along with getting to know your body and to eat God's food which grows out of the ground.

These foods rebuild your immune system, your white blood cells, clean your red blood and arteries, rejuvenate your kidneys, bladder, and pancreas, clean your colon, and release toxins from the exterior body and brain. They also restore the immune system, equilibrium, electricity, enzymes, coenzymes, minerals, vitamins, blood pressure, sugar, cholesterol, helps asthma, lupus, memory, sight, allergies, impotency, prostate cancer in men, balance women's total hormone structure, and control many long term hormone problems, menopause, and hot flashes.

They also give a woman everything that she needs to give birth to a perfectly healthy baby, help with menstrual pains, puts back all the nutrients which a woman loses during her time of the month, and works as a total healing source of life!

This book will show you which foods to eat and how cancer begins with bad bacteria growing into what the medical industry calls cancer cells.

In my vision, cancer is simply bad bacteria in its 2nd, 3rd, and 4th stages, with airborne toxic buildups in the body destroying white blood cells which have a low amount of oxygen, in addition to breaking down your red blood cells and your immune system. Bad, dying cells and dead cells hanging out in your body cause you cancer and many other blood related diseases.

The answer is to rebuild the immune system and put the oxygen back into the white blood cells, clean the red blood cells and destroy the bacteria, the toxins, the dead and dying cells.

"Hand a man or woman a fish and feed them for a day, teach a woman or man to fish and you feed them for life."

Start off by drinking one half cup of GRAPE SEED OIL. Drink one full cup of **Brown APPLE CIDER VINEGAR. Vinegar Burns the Cancer;** it is God's Liquid Drano, and God's way of taking care of the cancer problem naturally, without using chemo or radiation. Wait about 20 minutes then drink about four glasses of water to flush out your system. The next step would be sending a six to eight once glass of **Pomegranate Juice** of Love to coat your and repair your kidneys, your bladder and your pancreas. Let the juice set in your system for about 3 hours. This is to protect these organs from the harshness of the vinegar. If you can't hold the vinegar down long, flush immediately with several glasses of water. Then flush your system down with water again.

The next step would be to get going with **The Three Kings** chapter in my book.

Start eating **Mustard Green Salads,** drink **Pomegranate Juice,** and eat **Bee Pollen** and **Hummus,** loaded with a lot of **Fresh Crushed Garlic** and all the **Wild King Salmon** that you can put down.

It is very important to keep your stomach lined with oil to protect your stomach lining from crappy foods and toxic poisons, maggots, worms, and so on. The vinegar (and sometimes garlic) will always continue to burn everything that is not good for your system, while allowing all other foods which are good and nutritious for the body to do their Godly and natural function.

In short, vinegar and oil guard the good food and beats up on the bad foods, while having them ready on your body's assembly line to be kicked out the door safely through your colon.

Consume each of these ingredients until you feel like throwing them back up - at that point you body has consumed all that it can take of that one item. I know that these ingredients are repeated three times for my readers and it is all in the spirit. One for the Father, one for the Son and one for the Holy Spirit. When you hear it three times it marks three spots across your brain, helping you make one step while God makes two.

This is my cure and vision through God of the basic steps of curing cancer with God's food. You must also read the entire book because there are many dos and don'ts that coincide with reaching this Godly and Successful Mission. All Praises to God!

When you use brown APPLE CIDER VINEGAR along with GRAPE SEED OIL, you preserve and pickle your body. If you are, for example, 40 years old, or whatever age you start to consume brown APPLE CIDER VINEGAR, you pickle your body. Your organs will now stop aging and they will not grow any older. In this case its 40 and your organs will stay this age as long as you continue my system of eating brown APPLE CIDER VINEGAR and GRAPE SEED OIL with your meals. Our bodies are designed to accept the vitamins in foods in a few different ways. Brown APPLE CIDER VINEGAR, mustard greens (raw and cooked), pomegranate juice, bee pollen, and fresh garlic will always attack cancer anywhere it finds and meet cancer in the body. The mustard greens, brown APPLE CIDER VINEGAR, and the garlic will travel to areas of the body and places in the brain that get rid of the cancer unknown to doctors because you can't see them with a microscope or scanners. My program is the best way to prevent diseases while simply having faith in God and eating his food. If you don't have faith in God then I cannot say that this will work 100% for you. **REMEMBER IT'S ALL ABOUT GOD!**

I have been living without doctors for thirty years and I am exactly the same size I was in high school, at 49 years of age today. Our bodies are our temples, which we must learn to love, understand and have a relationship with. In our daily lives we love 61 and have relationships with other people and other things. Now is the time to stop and make it perfectly clear to our own minds that we will have a true relationship with our body and stomach and the things we put in it and on it. **The big secret to curing cancer is knowing what foods stop the cancer, kill the cancer, and remove it safely from the body.**

# COME'ON WITH THE COME'ON AND START TALKING TO YOUR STOMACH

My vision from God and my Black/Cherokee Indian grandparents is one of the most important steps of this book. Once you have mastered this step everything else is downhill.

When I say Come' on with the Come' on what I mean is this - "Get with it, get inspired, kick your own self in the rear and get involved with talking to your stomach and your body as you would anybody else". Take a minute this morning when you wake up and say hello to your stomach and body, whether you say it out loud, or just in your head. Say I love you to your kidneys, your heart, and your brain. Start getting into communication with your stomach with the same energy you would use if you were trying to fall in love and have a relationship with someone else.

Remember, we pay attention to our hair, face, car, and our home. Now let us pay attention and communicate with our body. Consider it a little project that we do at home to show God thanks for the blessings of our wonderful bodies, while having faith that God's food will heal and nourish us. These foods all come from the ground.

I talk to my body and stomach even in my sleep and in my dreams. In our new home program or project (which ever you would like to call it), we must be very concerned about the food which enters our stomach. Everything that we eat or put into our body has to go somewhere. These foods, be it natural foods or manmade foods tampered with in the laboratories, will ultimately determine what happens to your body, by way of cause and effect.

In most cases, people generally have issues and problems with their health much later down the road. Sleeping, eating, and walking properly plays a major role in your life and health. On any day that you get a thought or notion to have grapes, a pickle, or banana, or maybe beans or a bag of peanuts — well, guess what! - This is exactly what your body is being depleted of! So don't just let that thought pop in and out of your mind in a split second. Hold that thought and stop as soon as possible and get your grapes, that pickle, banana, or milk and peanuts. By doing this you will notice a difference and a change for the better in your health. At the same time your user-friendly stomach is noticing that you are paying attention to it.

You are now on the right track. Today you get 100 points for having a good relationship and communication with your stomach. The stomach always sends signals to the brain when it wants something. We must take part in pushing personal matters aside, in order to pay closer attention to our body.

We pay attention to the person we are falling in love with. Now let's pay an equal or more time to our stomach! A person who eats and sleeps like this appears, to other people, like they have been working out all day, when they have not.

Try watching funny movies to relieve stress. Also try smiling sometimes when

you don't want to. All of these things which I
am talking about lower stress. Once you
have the stress lifted and your eating habits
have changed, you are half way home.
Doing this will heal most of your bodies
illnesses.

# MAKE FRIENDS
# WITH YOUR
# STOMACH AND GET
# READY TO RECEIVE
# THE GREAT
# RESULTS OF GOD'S
# BLESSINGS!

# YOUR SMART, USER-FRIENDLY STOMACH HAS A MIRROR INSIDE

We must learn how to become more user friendly with our stomach, so that our stomach can become user-friendly with us. We must also not get on a kick about dieting and taking vitamins, but instead we should simplify our minds and consider giving ourselves a program of various foods which are user-friendly to our stomach and our survival.

The more we do this, the more our stomach recognizes that we are in communication with it. As a result, the stomach acts as a mirror, in the way that when we give our stomach a good food source which it likes and needs, the stomach rewards us by healing the body, just as a mirror reflecting light.

If you could only see the picture of good food going into the body while the body turns on the switch "Automatic to Heal".

Then a receipt is sent to your brain saying blessings from God. Now look on the other side of the coin - when you put bad foods and substances into your body, your body's user-friendly system kicks on and an automatic switch says "Start Shutting the Body Down".

Now the bad foods get sent to various locations, just like a hit man being sent to a destination in your system to break you down, such as your pancreas. Let's just think about it. If your upper stomach cannot break up and digest the bad over-processed foods, neither can your lower stomach nor pancreas. So why pass the buck and push these problems to your kidneys and bladder by way of your pancreas?

You have now given cancer a personal invitation to void your system because this crappy food is not accepted anywhere in your body. Please remember that your stomach is much smarter than you think - it does not like strangers. You don't like strangers in your home or car, nor does your stomach.

Here is another example. In the body we only have friends and foe. The friends are entitled to come in, but the foe must hit the door. Try to imagine good foods in your 67 body fighting to heal you even when you are asleep. Now every time you put bad foods in your stomach is like taking down your own soldiers which are sent by God to protect you. You are now allowing the enemy, which in this case is crappy food, to conquer your Holy Temple, The Body!

God has blessed us with a user-friendly, "Automatically Healing Body", where we must be user-friendly and allow our system to function properly. When and if ever we try to trick our system, it simply and automatically makes us pay the cost.

When people start learning to eat like God's animals, then we would learn more about the healing of ourselves. Most animals, birds, and other life forms which God has created, only eat what is necessary, and when it is necessary to survive. Our health has a lot to learn from this. This is the theory that works best in health. This is also the theory that I use and the way that I have been living without doctors and pills for the last 30 years.

# LETTER OF HEALTH

I have been given a letter of health from my insurance company, which is a top, leading contender in the life insurance business - a wonderful company in business for over one hundred and fifty years. Their agents told me that the letter of health which was given to me was only given to a couple of women in the last 45 to 50 years, and to no men, and that this was the first time they had ever seen such a letter.

This letter stated that because of my blood test and all other tests, the company did not consider me at risk of getting any diseases of any kind for the next 3 years, and that I did not have to retest regarding upgrading my insurance policy for the next 3 years. I still have this policy and will always use this company to insure me and my family.

Understand that every time you upgrade a life insurance policy, the reputable and legitimate companies will retest you to make sure that you are having no additional health problems or diseases - most companies don't take risk.

The agents at this insurance company said that they had never heard of such a letter of health to anyone. So they called me in and asked me to sit down. In a very curious way they proceeded to ask me, "What do you eat, what do you put into your body?"

Oh, well, I gave them the whole story about what I ate. I eat nuts in the place of meat on many days for lunch, followed by 1 quart of soy milk, cranberry juice, or 100% grape juice. Pomegranate juice is also my favorite, and lots of mustard greens, garlic, vinegar, extra virgin olive oil, olives, GRAPE SEED OIL, lots of tomatoes, parsley and cilantro, many green herb seasonings, beans of all types, sea salt, bee pollen, honey, maple syrup, and no white bread, no white sugar, no white grease. I only eat when I am hungry and no other times. When my brain says I'm full, I stop and put the rest away for later.

# NEVER DIET

Never diet to lose weight - it adds stress to the brain. Diet is a four-letter, bad word, which is marketed to the American public to make billions of dollars, and seldom solves the problem.

The American public needs to be deprogrammed. Eat using my program, which is God's way of healing and nourishing the body. Once your body starts to heal, losing weight will come as an additional bonus from God as a result of you having faith in God's food!

# NEVER DIET

Diet is a four letter word that has been one of America's largest marketing tools concerning the area of health. America needs to be deprogrammed from the word *diet.* The simple serious thought of the word diet causes a liquid bacterial fluid which can grow into cancer.

The world of dieting is extremely complicated and no one ever gets it right for each individual because of the different structures of everyone's body - their molecular system. It is much simpler to follow God and his animals' program of eating. Animals for the most part only eat what is necessary, when it is necessary, and leaves food behind when they are full. Most animals don't carry a doggie bag of food home.

We need to learn to not overeat because we see a large portion of food, or learn to turn food down when someone invites you to dinner and you're not hungry but simply trying to please that person. Eat to fill your hunger pain then stop; don't eat to get full.

The stomach is about the size of a grapefruit and we stretch it the rest of the way. Try to only eat on the days and at times when your body needs food. Your stomach will always let you know.

Example: some days I don't eat because my body feels no hunger, or I may not eat breakfast or lunch that day. On these days and times, your body takes a rest from food, while allowing our Godly, high-tech, user-friendly system to heal.

Do not eat within 3 to 4 hours of going to bed. Also do your best to get proper sleep as the animals do. Animals don't give up sleeping to catch a late night show. Getting proper amounts of sleep will allow calories to burn and food to digest; it also gives your immune system a chance to rebuild the way God has planned.

There are many days when I eat only once a day. When you eat the proper foods, it sends a signal to your brain that you need fewer nutrients to run the body as a result. You don't get as hungry and you subconsciously start losing weight without knowing it. At the same time, you don't have excess food left in your body that overworks your bladder, kidneys, and pancreas.

We sometimes overload our ice boxes with food that we have to throw away; well, it's not that easy for your stomach to throw food away. You see, it is not at all about dieting, but eating on a program which works for your body.

The food we eat is very important; also talking and listening to your stomach. Our grapefruit-sized stomach does not like being stretched, pushed out of shape, and forced to handle more than necessary. You will not overload your car with people because you can't drive safely. So why do you overload your stomach which helps drive your body!

Remember, what you see with your eyes and what your stomach actually need are two different worlds apart.

**There are many people who I have helped heal with the power of God's food. I may not choose to advertise these people's names personally. I feel that this type of advertising and marketing feeds the ego of man. God heals and does not advertise who.**

Therefore I feel no need for praise, or to advertise whom I have helped. As a servant, I only feel the need to help heal God's people. This is my way of showering the world with love, while I am here.

# MAKE FRIENDS WITH YOUR BODY AND GET READY TO RECEIVE THE GREAT RESULTS OF GOD'S BLESSINGS!

Here's an example and point made once in this book and now made again. On any day that you get a thought or a notion to have a grape, a pickle, a banana, beans, or a bag of peanuts. Well guess what, that is exactly what your body is being depleted of.

# TAKING NAPS

Taking naps regularly certainly helps the immune system to rebuild, relieve stress, and lowers blood pressure. The only time your body truly heals 100% is during your sleep. Please keep that in mind any time something ails you.

Once you have become user-friendly with your stomach and eating, you will be able to rest or sleep ten times easier. You will began to dream again as you did back in high school. While in a good dream, you will lose weight in your sleep. Some nights I lose 2-3 pounds in my sleep during a dream. The reason being is that when you are dreaming, you are in motion doing something or going places. The actions of your subconscious mind cause you to burn fat. I sometimes dream four dreams a night, wake up, use the restroom and then go back to sleep in 30 seconds and back into the same section of the same dream.

When I was a little boy, my mother would make my sister and I take naps. In today's world people don't do that much anymore; they don't force their children to take naps. As a result this is one of the many reasons why children are growing up with such bad health. Some children whose bodies require naps don't reach their natural height that they would have grown if they had naps on a regular basis, or their bodies and organisms on the inside don't fully mature.

Fully matured organs work at 100% unless injured through blood passage or other. But organisms that have not fully matured cause many health complications that may later cause disease. When this individual grows old in age, he or she may have severe health issues.

A baby or child who does not take regular naps stands a strong chance of having a weak immune system, growth issues (internally and externally) in body mass and height. It also affects the child's ability to learn, read, and their control of behavior due to different sections of the child's brain not fully being developed due to lack of sleep. It is very important that everyone takes a nap, from 1 day old to 125 years old.

On one of my vacations in Madrid, Spain, I was introduced to taking naps on a much broader scale. Everyone there was taking naps they called it siesta; this took place twice a day when I was in Spain. The kids at school would have sleeping cots in the classrooms. They had a much longer school day because taking naps was a part of their curriculum. You would see men working on high rise buildings come down to go take a nap. The city looked like a ghost town during siesta time. Mainly doctors and surgeons kept on working.

Sleeping helps to rebuild all active and inactive cells in your body, when your food supply is being properly supported by a balance of nutrients and vitamins. I am really grateful to God for teaching me the art of taking a nap. No wonder the people of Spain live so long and look so beautiful.

Now let's talk about how taking naps relates to your brain - clearing your thought process while allowing you to make the right decision as to when and when not to eat. Please understand this is not a diet, but a program in which your mind and body together work as a team.

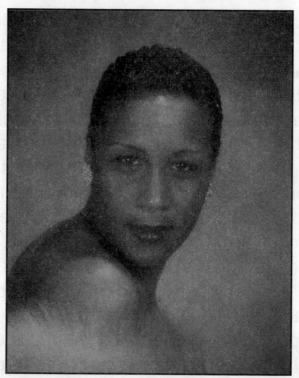

## In Memory of My Loving Sister Joyce B. Harris

My loving sister died of a very rare disease called T. T. P., a rare white blood cell disease which doctors knew very little about. The white blood cells quit making their own plasma, and blood surfaces to the top of the skin, and it is very fatal. Joyce, my sister, is one of the main reasons for my search for a food that would cure blood related diseases.

# WHITE BLOOD CELLS

Your white blood cells are very important in the fight of cancer. Through the progressing stages of cancer, the white blood cell are dying and breaking down. This breaking down and dying of the white blood cells, along with a rapid decline and breakdown in your immune system, is what makes cancer such a serious health issue.

There are many other diseases which follow these symptoms and kill at a much faster rate than cancer. One in particular I would like to talk about is called (TTP) Thrombotic Thrombocytopenic Purpura - a rare white blood disease. When my sister passed on to Heaven, there were only 5 cases of this disease in the state of Missouri and 50 cases in the state of California back in the early eighties.

TTP, simply described, is where the blood cells break down - quit making their own plasma. They break down and the blood vessels burst; you can see the blood rise to the highest level of the skin without out coming out, this was visually what I saw in my sister's final hour here on earth. She died within 10 days of going into the hospital.

She went into the hospital with headaches, thinking they were from menstrual problems. Joyce had ten doctors work with her every day. Surgeons communicating from country to country via computer and satellite, due to this being such a rare disease.

The Red Cross donated the blood for a total and full blood transfusion each day. The white blood cells will not accept artificial plasma - they must create their own or we die. Doctors still today don't have an answer to rebuilding the white blood cells properly, and in a Godly and natural way. This is why my quest to find the perfect natural food for rebuilding the white blood is so strong in my heart.

The breaking down and loss of white blood cells, and a low immune system, are two of the main symptoms of cancer. We must rebuild our white and red blood cells and our immune system to properly combat cancer. When your white blood cells start dropping off and dying, you will need to immediately rebuild them by feeding the blood oxygen.

The best way to naturally get oxygen into the blood is by eating green leafy plants, herbs or vegetables. **Here in my book I feature the Mustard Green as the top of the line source of oxygen - it rebuilds and rejuvenates. The mustard seed is the least of all seeds, which grows to be greater than all herbs, says the Bible, and that's why my faith is in the mustard seed. It is God's comparison to his kingdom. Mark Ch. 4, verse 30:32.** I have been eating them raw now for the past 25 years; before I only cooked them.

If you cook the mustard green in water, sea salt, and garlic, they work wonders through your digestive tract, and very well throughout your colon as a super natural cleanser. The oxygen from the raw mustard green will send oxygen to your blood right away, and also to all of your upper respiratory system and throughout your brain.

It rebuilds blood cells everywhere it goes. It also clears and unclogs your respiratory system, allowing a free-breathing passage for asthma patients to get that first breath of fresh air through their lungs and passage. Be it young or old, it helps sleep disorders!

One of my friends who is an asthma patient for many years tried the mustard green, after I showed him the passage about the mustard green in the Bible. His eyes turn red for about thirty seconds from the spicy mustard green. Then he began to say that he has not had a breath of fresh like that in years. Five minutes later he went and washed seven loads of clothes, and said that he had plenty of energy.

Natural 100% oxygen from the mustard leaf energizes the body and stimulates the brain. Doctors don't speak about it, nor does anyone in the medical industry speak of it. Doctors are not familiar with the full benefit of the mustard green and what is does because doctors don't use the Bible as a part of their malpractice.

**All the intelligence of the entire medical world does not add up to one mustard green leaf.**

Mustard greens have airborne active oxygen agents that microscopes can't fol83 low; they are far beyond the knowledge of doctors and scientists, traveling to unknown specific places in the body and your brain, healing faster than a stroke of lightning.

The mustard green is an amazing comparison of the healing power of God's kingdom! Basically, mustard greens lift you off your feet and get you going. When I eat my mustard green I feel like a king. I feed it to my child with the slightest inclination of a cold.

**If you eat my mustard green salad or mustard greens raw, it will stop a cold in its tracks. Try buying the Curly Leaf.**

Mustard greens and beans also stabilize people who have Acid Reflux. The manager of my local grocery store told me of the effect when he followed my instructions about eating--how it relieved his problems of Acid Reflux. Mustard greens help balance the immune system a great deal, to where it allows your body to now accept acid where it did not before.

Mustard greens also attack cancer cells, killing them, allowing the immune system to stand strong. My breakthrough information about the mustard green will be the center 84 of conversations in the medical industry once my book is released. Most doctors won't believe this, and most will debate this because it is not written in any medical books. God's food has a life time of healings that the medical industry will never totally understand, unless doctors start dropping their medical books and start picking up the Bible. This is why God sends his messenger/ servants to spread the word. Most doctors are not members of God's health program because of the medical industry's financial greed.

## God Has Made
## Us Our Own
## Doctors and Nurses
## Of Our Own Hospitals,
## Which Are Our Bodies.
## And God's Food
## Is Our Medicine.
## Trust in God And
## Have Faith!

# GOD'S SPIRIT
# SENDS GOD'S BLESSINGS,
# THROUGH GOD'S FOOD

Pomegranate juice also plays a major role in rebuilding the red and white blood cells. It works like an oil change in your car, but for the blood, the super high antioxidants in the pomegranate juice fight like soldiers in your blood line.

Pomegranate juice holds the highest level of antioxidants of all liquids you will find. It also helps vision - I see much clearer when I drink pomegranate juice. Pomegranate juice is also responsible for helping clear my memory of my life history, back to age 3 and 4, to write you this book. It, along with the mustard green, work together as team clearing and fighting the toxins in your brain, therefore allowing you to think clearer, and to restore your memory.

Pomegranate juice also rejuvenates God's clock in your brain, allowing your brain to run like a train on a track - full speed ahead - and totally wakes up the brain. God knows that his antioxidants do some amazing things.

Bee pollen also brings many amazing features to the white and red blood cells because bee pollen rebuilds your immune system and acts as two people, one on each arm, holding you up, or, in this case, holding up the white and red blood cells, helping them back on their feet.

Now here is the picture of a weak immune system. Bad microscopic bacteria, attacking and setting in the middle of crappy food, intestinal filth with more bacteria, toxins, salt, grease and sugar, grouping together like a gang plotting to break down your immune system while stealing your bloods oxygen.

The maggots in the red meat are trying to eat whatever nutrients you have left, and from small to large tape worms do the rest, waiting in line to eat the maggots, pulling the plug on your immune system. People, this is not the picture of a happy stomach. Guess what? Cancer uses your crappy food supply, after it has been broken down to its lowest state, to grow more cancer.

These creatures can't wait to lump you up and spread throughout your body and break down your white and red blood cells as they go. Cancer grows in lumps and spreads like wildfire, just waiting to take over your system rapidly!

Getting 1,500 mg of calcium or more a day in your system can also help your white blood cells rebuild your immune system and help stop the spread of cancer. 1500 milligrams of calcium a day and bee pollen will also help a woman to birth the perfect baby.

Some countries have over 1000 milligrams of calcium in the water, which is high in minerals. These people, on average, live to be well over 100 years of age.

Hopefully you get a clearer picture now of how microscopic creatures police your body and do you in. Try not to make your body work so hard to clean up all that mess; just keep it simple - don't diet, just eat the right foods, and take a walk 45 minutes after you eat.

I have seen men and women in Madrid, Spain walking at 12:30 am around midnight - the couple was about 90 to 95 years old, but their bodies looked young - maybe 40 to 50 years old. I remember saying to my cousin Clarence, who lived in Madrid at that time, "Man that old guy looks like he could go a few rounds with a young man in a boxing match and win." I had total respect for this couple walking hand in hand.

We followed them into an ice cream parlor and had some ice cream. When this man and woman spoke it gave me chills. It was one of the greatest adventures of my life seeing two people that old, that healthy, and in love. I couldn't wait to get back to America to tell people how so many people in Spain lived to be a very ripe old age and hung out at night - that blew my mind.

The Flamenco shows had 3 to 4 generations of very healthy families in one house. It was fantastic. The senior citizens had much more energy than the young people.

I also learned to drink one glass of wine a day for good health with my dinner.

Brown APPLE CIDER VINEGAR works as God's Liquid Natural Drano for the body. It cleans arteries, blood, helps to lower blood pressure, cholesterol, sugar, fights cancer, cleans the colon, washes kidneys, bladder, pancreas, takes mucus off lungs, kills bacteria, kills maggots and worms in the body, controls weight, and helps control allergies. Soaking your feet in vinegar controls fungus on feet which cause cancer; when applied to the scalp it clears dandruff. It seasons food, cleans bathrooms and heals a sore throat. And on and on!

**Dying blood cells, no oxygen to the white blood cells, low and high red blood cells, simply bad blood, blood clots, and a weak immune system are the reasons for most blood related disease, such as cancer and aids and leukemia and so on. This book will help you solve most of these problems.**

Many things I express to you in this book may be repeated. I do this intentionally, so that by the time you finish reading this book, the healing program is totally understood. If you are a cancer patient in pain, not feeling well, maybe you have missed an important part in one chapter or another. Well, don't worry; you will pick it up in the next chapter. Remember, this book was written for you. This way God's blessings will flow through me unto you without fail.

# Your Ice Box
# Is Now
# Your Medicine Cabinet

# THREE TINY STEPS
# TO
# SECURING YOUR HEALTH

Ladies and gentlemen, once again I am not a doctor, but simply a Modern Day Food Medicine Man, and a servant in a Godly way! And a good cook too. I don't do any healing at all! You and God do! I simply show you how by these 3 easy steps:

1. Love God.

2. Your faith in God's food to heal and nourish your body

3. Your faith and love of yourself, and also your will and determination to live.

God has blessed me with the gift of spreading the message of How to Heal the Holy Temple, which we call our body, by eating God's food. I am the little boy who was called the Miracle Boy back in the mid fifties in St. Louis by his doctors, family and friends, church people, and from everyone in the neighborhood, or anyone, who had ever heard my story.

Old people and young people would always say to me in earlier days, "Boy it's a miracle that you are alive."

The church people would say "God has something special that he wants you to do in life".

Other people would say that God made me a miracle; "That boy has a special gift!"

Many of the people who have tried my Cooking Secrets have experienced very fast results.

**This is what *"Home Cooking to Cure Cancer"* will help do for you:**

    Cleanse Colon,

    Reduces   Colon   Rectal   Cancer,
           Prostate, Lung and Breast
           Cancer, Cancer of the Pancreas,
           Helps Diabetes,

    AIDS,

    Lowers Blood Pressure,

    Regulates Blood Pressure,

    Kidney Failure,

    Bladder Failure,

    Asthma,

    Lupus,

Clearing Allergies,
Narcoleptic Problems,
Relieving Sleep Disorders,
Better Sleep,
Deep Dreams,
Losing Weight,
Regulate Bowel Movement,
Clearing Bumps and Facial Skin
    Irritations,
Clearing Arteries and Blood Vessels
    that Cause Heart Attacks,
Restoring Oxygen to the Blood,
Rejuvenating Blood Cells,
Preserving Organs,
Restoring the Body,
Increasing Life and Overall Health,
Totally Rejuvenates the Brain.

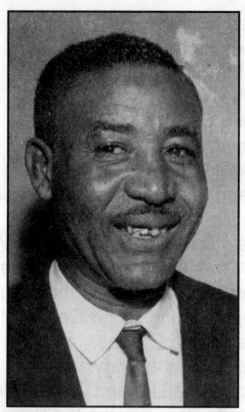

My Grandfather Robert B. McCallum

This is the man who inspired me to study the Mustard Green by reading the Bible when I was 7 years old. Mark Chapter 4 verses 30 – 32. My grandfather's dad was a Black/Indian Medicine Man. Robert's mother is Lu Nora in the beginning of the book. His mother died when he was 2 years old. His story is next.

# THE DOCTOR GAVE MY GRANDPA 24 HOURS TO LIVE

Not long ago my grandfather's doctor in the ICU ward of the VA Hospital told me to be prepared for the worst. He sat me down and said that my grandfather's kidneys had shut down and were not functioning at all, and that only the kidney machine had been keeping him alive at his ripe age of 89. The doctor said there was nothing left that he or the VA hospital could do, and he had given up.

My grandfather's body was very fragile from past surgeries. The doctor stated that I should start making preparations because he did not expect my grandfather to be alive the following day. After hearing this I decided to take over with prayer and the power of God's food.

I asked my grandfather's doctor if he would instruct the nurse to put pomegranate juice in my grandfather's feeding tube. I told him that I would buy it and take it to the hospital.

The doctor said that he did not think that would work.

Then I replied that my grandfather's dad was an Indian medicine man, and that I had inherited his gift, so please give him the juice to keep him alive.

The doctor at first looked at me in disbelief. He shook his head and said, "Young man, I know you have your grandfather's best interest at heart, but I don't think home remedies are going to work in this situation. I'm sorry to say your grandfather will expire by tomorrow, so be prepared." The doctor then also said, to satisfy me and my family, that he would instruct the nurse to put the pomegranate juice in the feeding tube. So the doctor eventually went along with my program after I had forced the issue.

I told the doctor that the family always has the last say. My dad, a VA hospital administrator, had always taught me that! I proceeded to ask the nurse to call me when she noticed a change in my grandfather's kidneys after giving him the pomegranate juice through his feeding tube, and she agreed to do so.

Twenty-four hours later the nurse called me and told me that my grandfather's kidneys had started working and the old man was doing fine. She stated that he released 3 quarts of urine within 24 hours. These were the same kidneys that the hospital said were shut down, and that my grandfather would die.

I jumped for joy and screamed "God's medicine is good - all praises to GOD."

The nurses in the ICU were totally amazed with my grandfather's outcome and wanted to know more about my cooking and food secrets for their own personal health.

I had also helped my grandfather with an asbestos problem, which he acquired while working for Firestone Rubber Company. Asbestos in the body also leads to cancer over a period of years. He was stirring 100% asbestos in the rubber to make tires with no protective gear for 45 years, and was involved with one of America's largest class action suits against Firestone/Bridgestone Rubber Company.

My food and health program helped him to survive this severe illness. His stomach would blow up where he looked like he was pregnant; he would also bleed through his private area, had dizziness and many other complications.

# God
# Has Made
# Us Our Own
# Doctors and Nurses
# Of Our Own Hospitals,
# Which Are Our Bodies.
# And God's Food
# Is Our Medicine.
# Trust in God And
# Have Faith!

# BLACK INDIAN MEDICINE MEN

Well, that's me; my heritage goes back to early American native black Indians. We are today a forgotten tribe and proud group of Christians that most Americans have never heard of.

America, throughout history, has made special efforts to not acknowledge the early American Black Indians. Trust me, it is a very cold feeling to know that your culture is not recognized as a civilization in a country which our own forefathers and mothers helped build, and also were the inventors and pioneers of early American medicine. Settlers at this time knew nothing of survival in this county called America.

Neither were we recognized in school history books as a civil group of people within the American society, who had numerous and countless home remedies which healed the body.

The Native Black Indians in the beginning were Black African slaves who ran away from their masters into the woods, and became friends, settled, and mixed with the Indians. They also fought in wars with Indians as blood brothers. These Black Africans mixed with the Indians and had children, and became the first natural settlers.

We lived our lives through wisdom, Black roots, the Indian spirit and Christian Godliness. My people were farmers, loggers and natural food healers. We believed in healing our bodies by the cooking of herbs and God's food to make our medicine. We used the woods and the forest as a full supply source for our food and medicine.

Each family used their own home just like you would use a hospital. Generally the dad or mom was the doctor. If someone got drastically sick we would get remedies from the tribal medicine man or from someone down the road in our community. Many Black Indian Medicine remedies were passed along through generations of families and to early American doctors and settlers who did everything that they could to make friends with these Black Indian Medicine Men in order to get their secrets.

My great-grandfather was a mix of Cherokee, Choctaw, Blackfoot, Redbone and African Medicine Man. My great Cherokee grandmother is one of my greatest inspirations of information and wisdom of health. I have been talking to her in the spirit for the past 30 years. I have never seen her in person she passed away when my grandfather was 2 years old.

I also find it amazing that I look more like my Cherokee Indian Grandmother than anyone in my entire family. We are without a question a team within the spirit. Now, today, you the people of America and other countries can learn the secrets of early American Native Black Indians and how we heal the body.

# THE
# MUSTARD GREEN IS
# ONE OF GOD'S
# GREATEST BLESSINGS
# TO HIS KINGDOM –
# WE MUST LEARN TO
# ACCEPT IT INTO OUR
# DAILY LIVES AND
# UNDERSTAND HOW IT
# RELATES TO THE
# SURVIVAL OF
# OUR HOLY TEMPLE,
# OUR BODY.
# HAVE FAITH IN THE
# MUSTARD SEEDS.

# THE THREE KINGS
# Mustard Greens,
# Bee Pollen,
# Pomegranate Juice

## MUSTARD GREENS

First we have the **Mustard Green** (cures diabetes, high blood pressure, blood sugar imbalance, and cholesterol). I put it first in line because it's the King of the Garden. The Bible states that the mustard seed is the tiniest seed, which grows to be the greatest of all garden herbs, vegetables.

Plants give off oxygen that we need to breathe, and we give them carbon monoxide - what they need to breathe. When we eat this mustard green, which is the greatest herb in the garden, it loads up our body with exactly what we need the most to fight cancer and to sustain life - "OXYGEN".

Cancer breaks down and eats away at our blood cells and immune system. The mustard green, king of the garden, helps to rebuild our white blood cells, red blood cells, and our immune system. It also fights hard to keep bad bacteria/cancer from coming back, and it cleans arteries.

Clean air, water, and blood inside our body's system are extremely vital to fighting all diseases, and it's hard for doctors to understand how to acquire this naturally.

We need oxygen in the blood - the mustard helps our blood create its own plasma. White blood cells must have natural plasma; if it does not create its own plasma, many diseases can take place and we die.

When my family eats mustard greens raw in a salad, we do not catch colds! I make a very small salad and give it to my child whenever there is a change in weather. This keeps her immune system in check by simply going with the flow. Animals in the wilderness have systems that change and flow with the weather and so must we.

An example of how we should get into the flow. When you travel around town or through different states, countries, and through different climates, or the weather just seems to be unstable and very unpredictable where you live, this is the time to eat more of these foods we are talking about. This is how we keep our stomach and system regulated to one another.

Spicy, which the mustard greens are, also help clear the lung passage, attacks mucus, helps all upper respiratory problems, helps with sleep disorders by giving you energy to stay alert, along with fighting inflammation and allowing free breathing, which makes it an excellent idea for asthma patients to eat mustard greens raw or in a salad.

Mustard greens when cooked clean out your digestive system and colon; it is one of God's natural forms of detoxifying the body.

The mustard green can also be blended in a fruit drink, with soy milk, pineapple and banana and orange juice. Pop in two curly leaf mustard leaves and blend.

---

## SHOPPING: WHERE DO I GO?

I buy GRAPE SEED OIL at the International stores. They also have the garbanzo beans, the olives, and a large selection of fresh herbs. These stores are without a doubt the key to life. And some local stores produce department. Watch out, DO NOT get foods which have been coated (wax, chemicals, etc), STAY AWAY from anything "FLAVORED", this means NOT REAL food. Check labels carefully.

**I REPEAT, I REPEAT NEVER EAT RED MEAT IF YOUR GOAL IS TO CURE CANCER OR ANY OTHER DISEASE!**

**Red meat makes the cancer grow fast. This guide book shows which foods to choose to fight the spread of cancer, which is the solution in my program of curing cancer.**

# BEE POLLEN

Bee pollen is Gods ultimate food source. It is the most complete food source on the planet. Bee pollen is loaded with more than 134 different nutrients. Today's high-tech doctors and pharmacology do not have a clue of the many secrets that Mother Nature's bee pollen holds.

Bee pollen is the most powerful source of vitamins, minerals, enzymes and coenzymes, and nutrients on the planet. It also has amino acids, proteins, globulins and peptones. Bee pollen has a host of healing capabilities. Here's what it does.

1. Bee pollen fights cancer by rebuilding your immune system to maximum strength and balance

2. It stimulates the brain, helps with memory, helps recall thoughts, helps headaches, helps you to have a good night's sleep, opens your subconscious state of mind allowing you to dream. An overall powerful food.

3. Bee pollen has been successfully used to cure all allergies due to all sorts of things. Bee pollen has also helped me in the area of allergies to dogs and cats. I

have noticed that some animals I use to quickly walk by; I now tend to look them straight in the eye and talk to them for a little while.

4. Bee pollen gives you energy. Bee pollen and bee honey are the only 100% natural stimulants allowed by the Olympic committee. Mohammed Ali, the famous boxer, would take bee honey and pollen before each fight. This is why he would say "float like a butterfly, sting like a bee." With bee pollen, your 12-hour days at work are now a breeze.

5. Bee pollen helps the relationships of people who are married by bringing back their youth. It is God's natural arousing stimulant for potency. Bee pollen helps make men potent and women fertile. If you are a married man or woman losing your relationship due to impotence, this, in most cases, solves the problem.

6. Bee pollen puts back all the vitamins, nutrients, replaces a man's hormonal structure, and also balances a woman's hormonal structure, sending signals to her brain that balances her time of the month. This helps to reduce

cramping, physical and mental pain, and a host of other female problems. It also helps the control of hot flashes and menopause.

7. After taking bee pollen for over 25 years, believe it or not, I will be skipping menopause and having no signs of it.

8. My brother gives small amounts of bee pollen to his dog and has noticed a much happier, vibrant, and energetic dog, with a beautiful coat of fur. His dog use to get sick and tired, but not anymore.

9. Bee pollen also helps Narcoleptic disease and all sleeping disorders. I have one of my friends taking bee pollen and he does not fall asleep while driving anymore.

10. Bee pollen, otherwise in biblical times known as manna, was mixed in the bread that the wise men ate on their journey of 40 days and 40 nights through the desert. This was all they ate and they were perfectly healthy by the end of the journey.

11. Bee pollen helps anyone who does not have the appetite to maintain a healthy diet. All minerals in bee pollen are present in a highly digestible and organic form necessary for the digestion of many

foods, functioning of glands, organs and nerves, and the balancing of blood, lymph, and aqueous and general metabolism system. Bee Pollen also contains active antibiotic substances, which destroys bacteria on contact. Bee pollen is useful in cases of stress and nervous endocrine system disorders due to its high content of natural B Vitamins. Bee pollen increases energy and mental alertness and is believed to slow down the aging process.

**Bee Pollen** is loaded with the nutrients:
**Vitamins** A, B-1, B, B-3, B-5, B-6, B-7, B-8, B-12, C, D, E, H, K, and vitamin PP.
**Minerals** Calcium, Phosphorus, Iron, Copper, Potassium, Magnesium, Silica, Sulphur, Sodium, Titanium, Zinc, Iodine, Chlorine, Boron and Molybdenum
**Proteins, Globulins Peptones and Amino Acids** Tryptophan, Leucine, Lysine, Isoleucine, Methionine, Cystin, Thresonine, Arginine, Phenylalanine, Histidine, Valine, Glutamic acid, Tyrosine, Glycine, Serine, Proline, Alanine, and Aspartic Acid
**Enzymes and Coenzymes** Disstase, Phosphatase, Amylase, Catalase,

Saccharas, Diaphorase, Pectase, Cozymase, Cytochrome systems, and Succinic Dehydrogenase

Bees fly a 40-50 mile radius from the bee farmer's home and queen bee, and collect the pollen from the inside of flowers and plants and other sources of nature. When you eat the pollen you are eating your environment.

Bee pollen is better to take in the morning or before each meal if you need energy. Only take small amounts. Maybe start off with about 15 pellets in the morning and 15 in the afternoon. Never take within 4 hours of going to bed.

Each day that you feel no effect, increase the pollen a little more. The feeling you should get from bee pollen is that you are wide awake or very alert, that you have more energy than you ever had, that you don't get tired anymore in the middle of the day. You feel full with no thoughts of hunger. Bee pollen sends a signal to your brain that you have all the vitamins and minerals that you need, therefore causing you to not be hungry while you're subconsciously losing weight, by taking bee pollen on a regular basis.

Bee pollen does have some side effects, but they are controllable if you make sure that you don't take excessive pollen. Remember to start off with no more than 15 pellets - this is very important due to the ultimate concentrated strength of the bee pollen.

If you are fully blown with terminal cancer, take ¼ table spoon 3 times a day and work your way up each day. Please remember to gradually increase the pollen and never double the amount at any given time.

Kids under 12 years of age should start off with about 10 pellets and gradually go up.

These are the side effects; if you feel any of these symptoms, pull back and take less pollen, or stop until you have control of the amount you take in. I repeat it is extremely powerful.

If you feel stomach aches, itching, diarrhea, tightness of facial skin, the need to throw up, then you should take less pollen. If you are overweight you may take more than a thin person; if you eat out a lot at greasy restaurants then you may take more than a person who eats healthy.

You can find bee pollen at your local farmers' markets or wherever the farmers bring their goods to town. Some health food stores carry it, but make sure that the pollen you buy comes from your state, or within 200 miles of where you live. It works best when it is closest to where you live.

Try to buy it unpasteurized - pasteurization is a process which kills 20% or more of the nutrients of the pollen. It is best to buy it from a bee farmer, fresh.

**I REPEAT AND MUST SAY AGAIN - Do Not Take more than** ½ teaspoon of bee pollen at the beginning. Start off with 5-15 pellets and work your way up to larger amount.

# Benefits of Pomegranate Juice

1. Pomegranate juice helps correct vision. I see clearly immediately.
2. Stimulates the brain
3. Restores memory
4. Fights cancer
5. Cleans and enriches your blood
6. Helps glaucoma
7. Breaks up toxins and pollutants in the brain and throughout the body
8. Helps aneurisms
9. Helps Alzheimer disease
10 Restores kidneys
11 Restores your bladder
12 Restores the pancreas
13 Helps your blood to flow
14 Helps to detoxify and clean arteries
15 Helps restore your equilibrium
16 Helps you to become more alert
17 Opens your subconscious mind, allowing your brain, on a daily basis, to have open and creative thoughts, taking your mind anywhere you want to go.

# POMEGRANATE JUICE

Pomegranate is the Third King, and it really deserves a high ranking as being one of the world's greatest fruits and the healthiest liquid drinks you will ever find.

Pomegranate has the highest levels of antioxidants of all liquid drinks. When you drink pomegranate juice there is no faking as to whether you had a health drink or not. It has more antioxidants that cranberry juice, grape juice, blueberry juice, or blackberry juice.

Pomegranates are one of the first five crops ever, along with figs, dates, olives, nuts, and grain about 3000 years B.C. in the area of Jericho. Some scientists believe it originated in Persia, and it's also seen in Turkey, India, North Africa, and Iran.

Pomegranate juice is a very good cancer fighter because of its Polyphenol Antioxidants. Antioxidants are cancer cell busters.

This juice was the main health drink of kings and queens. Over 2,500 years ago kings would have their servants gather up all the pomegranates and store them for the king and queen only. The people were not allowed to have a drop of this juice in most countries in those days.

Pomegranate juice has always been a sign of good health and is told to be a great preserver of life. They say that people who drink pomegranate juice will live forever. King Tutankhamen, better known as King Tut, was known to have put pomegranate seeds in his tomb, mixed in with his jewels, in hopes of preserving himself to come back in the afterlife.

Pomegranate seeds were also used to line the robes of Catholic priests in the old days.

It also helps to break up the polluted toxins you breathe in the air, refreshes your lungs and upper respiratory area, and helps blood circulation in legs.

# TURMERIC

Turmeric is a member from the ginger family and is used in many herbs and spices and used mainly as a food coloring.

Turmeric heals cuts and bruises. Helps your kidneys, bladder, pancreas, and lowers blood pressure to your heart. Turmeric is used in many herbs and spices, popcorn chicken, and curry powder. Turmeric helps to relieve strokes, Alzheimer and aneurisms.

Helps fight colds, helps with all skin diseases such as melanoma, fungus and rashes. Has reduced and got rid of inflammation throughout the body.

Turmeric is the most perfect rejuvenator of the facial skin cells and a great face mask.

Stir one Tablespoon of Turmeric in a cup with 5 Tablespoons of GRAPE SEED OIL and leave on your face for 25 minutes. Then steam it off. If you still have the orange color in your skin put brown APPLE CIDER VINEGAR on a cotton swab and swab your face with brown APPLE CIDER VINEGAR. TUMERIC terminates and disposes of worms, parasites and maggots, by the use of its drying affect.

I put as much TURMERIC in my food as possible every day, without changing the taste. Turmeric is 100% good for your body.

India, South Asia and the Middle East have been using TURMERIC as a AYURVEDA and Naturopathic medicine for thousands of years.

Turmeric, when used with GRAPE SEED OIL will preserve and coat your internal organs. This increases cell rejuvenation and lets your blood move at its full potential. This also allows your blood to use its own defense system to fight off disease. Turmeric stops ALL cancers all over the whole body. Stops mucus, and puts an end to Candida before it turns into cancer.

Boil turmeric and make 3 cups of tea a day to avoid and terminate breast and other cancer.

For gum disease brush your teeth and gums with turmeric at least twice daily. Turmeric is a natural fluoride for your teeth.

# GRAPE SEED OIL

**GRAPE SEED OIL** contains only essential goods fats that the body does need and none of the saturated bad fats (the ones we don't need). Studies have shown that GRAPE SEED OIL has a unique ability to raise HDL cholesterol (the "good" cholesterol), while lowering LDL cholesterol (the "bad" cholesterol) and triglycerides. (This reduces the risk of cardiovascular disease and impotency.) Also has valuable antioxidants, a strong source of vitamin C (more than Olive Oil) and vitamin E, three times the vitamin E of olive oil.

GRAPE SEED OIL has Omega 3, 6, 9 with seven times MORE essential fatty acids, such as Linoleic acid, (also known as Omega 6) than any other oil.

GRAPE SEED OIL never gets hotter than 400° F therefore no toxic smoke and is reusable after cooking. Olive oil becomes toxic and poisonous when you see it start to smoke.

GRAPE SEED OILS are NOT hydrogenated. GRAPE SEED OILS are the best because: NO sodium, NO trans-fat acids, NO cholesterol, and NO preservatives (like BHT or TBHQ).

This makes GRAPE SEED OIL the perfect Oil for preparing healthy hot and cold meals. GRAPE SEED OIL is the best oil in the world. Lubricates joints to prevent arthritis, protects the stomach lining from being eaten up by cancer. PREVENTS: ALL AILMENTS, cancer, strokes, high blood pressure, high cholesterol, Alzheimer's, ADD, ADHD, aids, diabetes, hair loss, Parkinson's disease, SIDS, colic, wrinkles, stretch marks, prevents hair loss and stimulates hair growth on your head, stops internal bleeding, shrinks varicose veins, prevents lice and is naturally safe for children.

Unclogs, reinforces and strengthens the internal/external walls of veins, arteries, capillaries, and all organs. Makes blood flow freely. Increases oxygen to the brain. Rebuilds your blood cells.

Restores digestive system, colon and bowel track and clears path to the lungs which increases oxygen breathing capacity. Increases male potency and female fertility to conceive a healthy, complication free, baby.

Removes fat tissue which reduces your weight and odors out of your bowel movement. Moisturizes, cleans and shines your face and skin, and all your leather, including your dress shoes for Church.

**PREVENTS, STOPS, RESTORES, REBUILDS and HEALS EVERYWHERE, IN ON AND AROUND YOUR BODY.**

Promotes better vision, and promotes longevity of life. Most of all makes you feel like a child all over again.

GRAPE SEED OIL heals cuts and bruises, rashes and all skin irritations for your dog or cat or any animal.

GRAPE SEED OIL will Remove arthritis. GRAPE SEED OIL heals internal/external bleeding for humans and animals.

**GRAPE SEED OIL** is one of Gods greatest gifts.

*EVERY AREA OF THE BODY IS ASSISTED BY THE MUSTARD SEED.*

*SWALLOW 3 TEASPOONS A DAY FOLLOWED BY WATER OR JUICE.*

*PUT MUSTARD SEEDS IN ALL YOUR FOOD: SOUP, SALADS, BEANS, JUICES etc.*

*CHEW THE MUSTARD SEED FOR MIGRAIN HEADACHES, or ANY PROBLEMS IN THE THROAT or BRAIN.*

The mustard seeds are one of God's greatest wonders.

MUSTARD SEEDS INCREASE THE BODY'S OXYGEN SYSTEM WHICH STRENGTHENS THE IMMUNE SYSTEM TO PREVENT DISEASE FOR THE WHOLE BODY.

# THE MUSTARD SEEDS

Your creator's ultimate spiritual, live molecular and active food source. Mustard seeds are God's way of moving oxygen, in God's scientific molecular electronic way, through the blood and all parts of the body, like a continuous wind of oxygen moving through your body. Scientists have a lot to learn about this seed.

My God has shown me how chewing this seed heals and removes: throat cancer, ovarian cancer, prostate cancer and all cancers, all sinus infections in the eyes and nose, clears the mucus anywhere in the body.

Mustard Seeds remove, prevent and stop migraine headaches, fibroid tumor or any tumor anywhere in the body, menstrual cramps, Alzheimer's, strokes, colds, fever, reduces your weight by sending oxygen through your colon forcing excess bowel to come out while cleaning your colon, removes feet pain even those who wear orthopedic shoes, sends oxygen through your blood to stop ADD, ADHD, SIDS, all cramps, blood clots, narcoleptic diseases. Strengthens male potency, increases fertility in a woman. REDUCES TUMORS ANYWHERE IN THE BODY

Stops tumors in dogs, cats and all animals, For full benefits of this incredible Mustard seeds, chew or at least swallow, 2-3 teaspoons every day, followed by water or juice. Consider mustard seeds your new pepper, good pepper that helps the brain.

DO NOT use black pepper. Black Pepper for many people causes heart attacks, sever headaches, high and low blood pressure, sends your sugar levels into a frenzy, also can cause scar-tissue on organs and inflammation in prostate, bowel track, kidneys, bladder, pancreas and anus, while clotting the blood causing a spasmodic inconsistent blood flow. A high pressured spasmodic blood flow can cause shock to your heart and cause you a heart attack.

Your veins, arteries, and capillaries are very thin, like paper, and can become damaged very easily. Many people, who have unhealthy organs and clotted blood, suffer severely when they eat black pepper. Black pepper can be a fast track to your funeral, because black pepper locks up your arteries. I don't eat white pepper either. I only eat the yellow, red, and orange peppers which grow up through the ground and very little of these. Peppers cause inflammation when the body has any issues.

Mustard seeds relax and unlock your blood and arteries, allowing your blood to have a constant normal flow. You can also eat mustard seeds in anything including your fruit juice, soup, salad or beans, put on your fish, chicken, turkey burger, add to everything.

Mustard seeds give you a super charge and a lot of energy for sports. They send oxygen to the brain, activating and charging your brain to a higher academic level of learning in grade school, high school or college.

Mustard seeds thicken your blood cells by rebuilding your white blood cells which in turn rebuilds your red blood cells.

Whenever you need to THIN your blood, just eat ginger and garlic raw or in juice DO NOT COOK.

NO ONE needs Cumidin to thin their blood. Cumidin slowly shuts down oxygen to the brain, killing brain cells and does massive damage to your body's organs, leaving poison in your feet and hands. Cumidin is a manmade disaster. When man puts poison in a human's body then for sure that man has lost control of HOW TO HEAL the body. Any patient who is given Cumidin is being terrorized: medically, sociologically and systematically! God will punish those whom make such poor intentional choices.

All the wise men around the world carried or carry seeds in a small pouch. The Bible and the Torah say the seeds shall be your meat, to every beast, to every fowl and to everything that crepeth across the earth. Gen 1 verse 29: the mustard seed is talked about in Mark Ch 4 verses 30-32.

The Chinese have been eating mustard seeds for over 2500 years. Mustard seeds are a famous French secret in cooking for hundreds of years.

America spends the most money for health care than any other country around the world but ranks number 37 in health care out of 151 countries and France ranks #1 in HEALTH CARE.

Mustard seeds are also the main secret ingredient in curry powder which is an Indian Ayurveda way of healing the body. Ayus meaning life and veda meaning science. FOR EXAMPLE: Curry powder lowers your blood pressure.

Mustard seeds contains: Protein, vitamin A, water, vitamin B1(thiamin), vitamin B2(riboflavin), vitamin B3(niacin), vitamin B6, vitamin B9(folate), vitamin B12, vitamin C, vitamin E, vitamin K, calcium, iron, magnesium, phosphorus, potassium, sodium, dietary fiber, zinc, manganese and are a very good source of selenium and omega-3 fatty acids.

Thank you God for all of this spiritual, electrical, oxygen which is carried within each and every seed.

There are 25 different variations of mustard seeds, some so small that they can barely be seen by the naked eye.

Mustard seeds replace toxic gas with good oxygen. This will make you release bad gas until all of it is removed from the body.

Relieves internal stomach problems that the medical field has no answer for. Thousands of people die every day sitting on the toilet from impacted stomach and bowel problems. Mustard seeds will stop the stomach pain, by relieving the pressure and bloating of the impacted stomach by releasing the bowel. Allows regular, frequent bowel movements.

Your clogged impacted stomach or viral infection has poisons, maggots or worms inside. Mustard seeds will help you naturally release fat, poisons, toxins, maggots and worms which reduces your weight. NOTE: A very small number of people initially may experience temporary bloating, throwing up or have large or frequent bowel movements.

For some people, mustard seeds go through them and out the bowel due to internal stomach lining problems, leaky gut syndrome or a very nervous system. If seed continues to come through, chew the seeds and consume 2-3 ounces of GRAPE SEED OIL a day. Drink or put in your food, till stomach lining repairs itself in 2-3 days.

# THE THREE WHITE
# KNIGHTS OF
# CANCER

The Three White Knights of Cancers are "Cancer's Army". The Three White Knights are Sugar, Salt and Grease. All three of these guys help cancer grow in a big way; they clot your blood, making problems for your arteries, your colon, your heart and organs.

If we were to name a fourth and fifth White Knight they would be Bacteria and Stress. In the place of sugar use honey, 100% molasses, maple syrup, or 100% raw sugar from the cane that has not been treated or pasteurized.

Raw honey is the best - it has the most nutrients. In the place of salt use sea salt. Do not use sea salt that includes the word iodized or any words similar to iodized. It will lump up and clot your blood. In the place of mayonnaise or grease use GRAPE SEED OIL. GRAPE SEED OIL adds vitamins and nutrients to your food that have been used for over 3,500 years and since the beginning of time. The grapes and olives were of the first foods God placed on earth. This is what being healthy is all about.

They also put a protective coating on your stomach walls and lining. Your stomach lining is very important to the body. It acts like a storage casing for your food, allowing proper digesting of your good food, and it protects you from what I call a caravan of microscopic attackers such as bacteria maggots, worms, and so on.

The lining is basically a force field in your stomach which helps protect you from stomach flu's - diseases in your stomach and other organs. To get 100% use of this force field you must put in 100% of God's food. Replace the bacteria with a regular program of eating natural foods and include meals from my cook book which include GRAPE SEED OIL, brown APPLE CIDER VINEGAR, garlic, sea salt, mustard greens - raw, cooked, and juiced - also radishes, green herb seasonings, curry, onions, peppers, and lemons. These items send nutrients to the body while breaking down fat.

The GRAPE SEED OIL sends this fatty dissolved mass, and other unwanted body waste, out through the colon and into your toilet without you knowing it. They send signals to the brain that the body is satisfied and you lose the thought of hunger. You can find these items in your local food stores and health food stores.

Regular salt will clot your blood, destroy your vessels by not allowing your blood to filter itself nor accept nutrients, harden your veins, and give you a heart attack. Sea salt, on the other hand, is good for you.

In the old days it was used for medicine as an antibiotic. American soldiers in past wars throughout history would impact their wounds with salt, after it had been shot off or cut off, to keep from dying. Early American Black Indian farmers would castrate the male mules because they did not want to work otherwise, and would use salt to immediately heal the wound.

Mahatmas Gandhi, a great man, started an uprising revolution because England was invading India and would not allow the people of India to extract the sea salt from the sea. In those days the Indian people used the salt as a medicine and antibiotics to heal the body. The people of India could not afford expensive medicines and there were thousands of people who were dying and needed medical care. Gandhi therefore starved himself until England would allow his people to extract the salt. England eventually gave up and changed their mind due to the wisdom and power of Gandhi's revolution, and allowed the people of India to extract the salt from the sea. The country of India won their victory. Everyone shouted with tears of joy because Gandhi had saved so many lives.

At 12 years old I studied the life story of Gandhi and believed very much in his words - he was a great wise man and mentor in my life as a young boy and a man. God Bless Mahatma Gandhi and his wisdom forever.

# FOODS THAT FIGHT
# CANCER GROCERY LIST

*"If you are in any way allergic or have symptoms due to these types of foods, consult with your doctor for alternatives"*

Mustard Greens, mustard seeds, GRAPE SEED OIL, Bee Pollen, Pomegranate Juice, Brown APPLE CIDER VINEGAR, Lemon, Garlic, Onions, Tomatoes, Olives, Green-Red-Orange- Bell Peppers, Curry, Rosemary, Original Chives, Ice Cajun Parsley, Sea Salt, Wheat Germ, Apples, Pineapples, Bananas, Cheese, Lebni, Garbanzo Beans, Sesame seeds, Tahini, Cilantro, Lentil Beans, Black Beans, Canned Beets, Broccoli, Cabbage, Baby Carrots, Soy Milk, Ginger, Peanuts, Almonds, Walnuts, Macedonian, Pecans, Mustard, Maple Syrup, Wheat Pasta, Red Wine, Corn Meal, Wheat Flour, Tofu, Portobello Mushrooms, Regular Mushrooms, Jalapenos Peppers, Lime, Wheat Pancake Mix, Bran, Wheat, Rice, Oat, or Rye Cereal, Potatoes, Tangerines, Cauliflower, Extra Virgin Olive Oil, Goat Cheese, Flat bread / Bible Bread, Hot Pepper Cheese, Mozzarella, Provolone Cheese, Parmesan Cheese, Eggs, Chicken Breast, Salmon, Ground Turkey, Red Snapper, Trout,

We must know about Gods food and how they work for us.

We must also get in touch with our stomach, our food and our body! Guess what - they work as a team!

**CONTROLLED BY GOD's FOOD**
**OUR MIND,**
**OUR BODY, AND**
**OUR SPIRIT.**

Let me help you learn how to cook to stop cancer cells while you eat to rejuvenate your blood cells back to life. Eat a Mustard Green Salad twice a day, for five days a week.

# HOME COOKING TO CURE CANCER *RECIPES*

# WE ARE THE DOCTORS and NURSES OF OUR BODIES, OUR HOSPITAL IS OUR HOME

# THE KEY AND SECRET TO LIFE IS GOD'S FOOD, WHICH IS GROWN FROM THE GROUND.

Remember, you are what you eat. God's foods, which are grown from the ground, are the only 100% natural way to stop the spread of cancer. Destroy the bacteria and cancer cells while rebuilding the white and red blood cells and immune system. Clean the body naturally.

# THE MUSTARD GREEN SALAD
## CURES DIABETES, HIGH BLOOD PRESSURE, BLOOD SUGAR IMBALANCE, and CHOLESTEROL

My recipe is quite simple.

1. A layer of chopped mustard greens on a plate.

2. Then slice three red tomatoes.

3. Put one layer of tomatoes over the mustard greens.

4. Add beets, olives, mushrooms, beans, tofu, cheese and any other vegetables you like.

5. Add garlic, ginger, or any other spices you like.

5. For your salad dressing, get three spray bottles. I buy spray bottles from the local 99¢ store. Fill one of the bottles with brown APPLE CIDER VINEGAR - use the brown vinegar only. Fill another bottle with GRAPE SEED OIL, and fill the third bottle with extra virgin olive oil. Spray your salad about ten times, heavy, with brown APPLE CIDER VINEGAR, and about ten or more times with GRAPE SEED OIL, extra virgin

olive oil or coconut oil. My first choice is the GRAPE SEED OIL.

Sprinkle your herbal seasonings, basil, rosemary, chives, parsley, cilantro, and oregano. You can also use garlic powder or fresh garlic; crush it up and put on the salad.

Get used to sprinkling your foods, I sprinkle my food every chance I get and have been doing this for several years. Sprinkling your food makes it very digestible, helping you to lose weight. Eat and enjoy!

To make a full meal out of this salad, add protein of choice, chicken breast cooked in lemon, or fresh wild king salmon cooked in parsley, garlic, basil and cilantro. Cook the protein, chicken or the salmon separately in a pan with GRAPE SEED OIL, brown APPLE CIDER VINEGAR, curry and always drink the juice from all of my recipes. The juices aid to heal and cure weight problems, cancer, cholesterol, sugar diabetes, kidneys, bladder, and the colon.

## MUSTARD GREENS

The mustard green leaf will send a large dose of oxygen to your blood, which will strengthen your white blood cells. The tomatoes are high antioxidants that help fight the spread of cancer.

It is very important not to throw away the stems of the mustard green. The stems are the best part and carry the largest amount of vitamins and nutrients. So take the stems in your hand, hold them together, and cut off the end of the stems every sixteenth of an inch. Put the stem on the top of the salad at the very end.

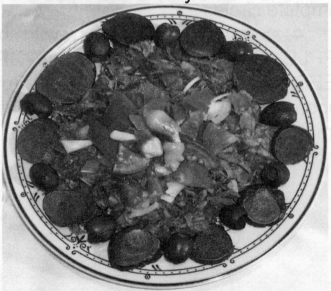

## MUSTARD BEET SALAD

# MUSTARD BEET SALAD

**1.** Get large plate, go 2 inches into plate and put one layer of chopped mustard greens in a circle.

**2.** Put a layer of chopped tomatoes in a center circle about 4 inches wide.

**3.** Now make a ring around the exterior of the mustard greens with one slice of beets then one black olive whole then continue around the salad with one beet one black olive until you have made a complete circle.

**4.** Spray 5 times each with brown APPLE CIDER VINEGAR and GRAPE SEED OIL or extra virgin olive oil. Put one spoon of mushrooms on top in center of tomatoes.

# QUEEN GREENS

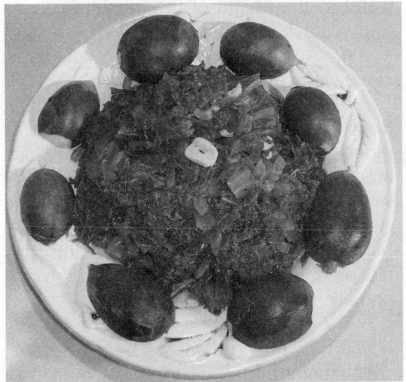

    **1.** Get 3 bunches of mustard greens – the curlier the leaf the better. Wash off the mustard leaf by running warm water, making sure that you wash off any insects.

    **2.** Cut the leaves about every 2-3 inches. Cut off stems of mustard leaf, but do not throw away - save for later.

    Shake water off leaves and place into pot.

**3.** Put water in the pot. Make the water ¼ the height of the mustard greens and spinach together.

**4.** Add 7 garlic cloves, cut garlic cloves into 1/3 pieces, place in pot.

**5.** Add 7 squirts of GRAPE SEED OIL from your spray bottle with the letter O taped or written onto the bottle (which stands for oil) and 5 squirts of apple cider vinegar, (the brown vinegar only, not the clear) with your V spray bottle.

**6.** Now chop up the stems into tiny pieces about 1/16 of an inch, place in pot, and stir.

**7.** Cook on low for about 3 to 4 hours – when the mustard greens become soft in consistency and easy to chew, then they are done.

# KING GREENS

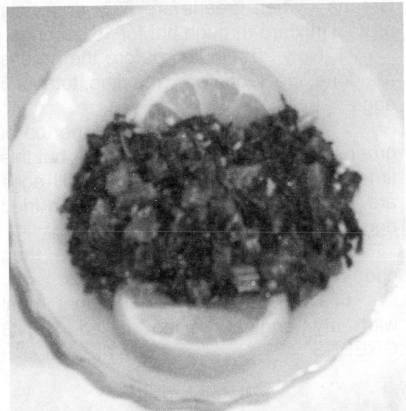

**1.** The same instruction as Queen Greens - spray frying pan with Grape Seed Oil.

**2.** Shake about 3 shakes of curry, 3 shakes of chives and 1 pound of ground turkey, mix, and cook in frying pan till ¾ done.

**3.** Put turkey in pot with Queen Greens - when greens are 80% done, stir protein mixture through pot for 15 seconds.

**4.** Now 20 minutes before the greens are done, crack one egg at a time, total of 5 eggs.

Drop and spread over the top of greens, break open the yellow yolk, but this time do not stir the greens, cook till eggs are totally done on top of greens to a fried egg consistency.

**5.** Let cool for about 10 minutes, then chop and stir the egg into the greens.

**6.** Now you have a full dinner meal with my original recipe called "KING GREENS".

# THE MUSTARD QUICHE

**1.** Get 1½ cup of wheat flower.

**2.** Add a few spoons of water, mix into flour to make a dough, add one pinch of sea salt and a pinch of baking power.

**3.** Roll dough flat and lay into 4-six inch baking pans.

**4.** Take one bunch of mustard greens and chop into small pieces. Place into a large bowl.

**5.** Add 3 eggs and

**6.** ½ cup of tofu, ricotta cheese or Lebni and

**7.** ½ cup of chopped mushrooms.

**8.** Now add 3 shakes of parsley, basil, chives, curry.

**9.** Now put everything into the baking pan with the dough - at least a four inch deep pan. Preheat oven at 325, put lid on pot or cover pan with aluminum foil, cook for 1 hour,

**10.** Take out of oven, let set for 20 min. Your lips should be starting to chomp by                                                              now!

# MUSTARD GREEN COOKIES / PASTRIES "MG SNACKY"

**1.** Spray pan first with GRAPE SEED OIL.

**2.** MIX together 1 Tablespoon GRAPE SEED OIL, 2 cups of brown flour, a pinch of sea salt, 1 egg and 1 teaspoon of water. Roll into a dough. Flour the board lightly and then Roll the dough into 4X4 inch squares and flatten out squares.

**3.** Chop up about 4 leaves of mustard green cut in to ½ inch pieces,

**4.** put greens on dough - enough to cover square.

**5.** Spread 1 spoon of Lebni on top

**6.** Pour 1 large tablespoon of honey over the top.

**7.** Put crushed almond, pecan, or cashew on top of honey.

**8.** Fold left and right edges to meet center, seal, and make pastry.

**9.** Bake for 30 min, let set for 10 min, and eat.

# SALSA "THAT'S SALSA"

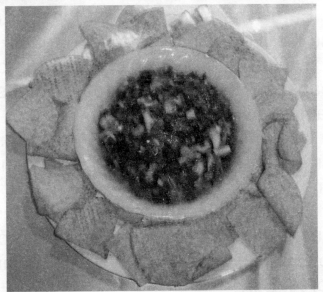

**1.** Cut up 2 onions and chopped green pepper if desired place in a large bowl. Cut up 4 large tomatoes into small pieces and place in bowl.

**2.** Cut up ½ bunch of cilantro into very tiny pieces, put in bowl. Squeeze in the juice of one lemon into bowl.

**3.** Add ½ cup GRAPE SEED OIL.

**4.** Add ¼ cup of gold apple cider vinegar, sprinkle 2 shakes of basil stir, and eat.

**5.** If you have NO heart problems, chop up and add small pieces of fresh green pepper.

# HUMMUS

Eat in the place of meat for your mind, and it will do wonders for your health.

**1.** Get 2 cans of chick peas (garbanzo beans).    Squash up into thick paste in plastic bowl.

Use only about 1/3 of the juice from the can which the beans were packed in, and stir.

**2.** Add 2 tablespoons of Tahini Sesame sauce, which is 100% sesame seed paste. You will find this at your international stores. Stir.

**3.** Add 4 cloves of fresh garlic, squashed up real fine.

**4.** Juice from 1 whole lemon into bowl.

**5.** Add 6 squirts of GRAPE SEED OIL and stir.

When done, it should be a thick paste, slightly creamy. Spread on pita or bible bread, or tear off a piece of lettuce leaf and use lettuce leaf to pick up and eat.

By eating a little bowl of Hummus, you will lose your hunger pain and totally nourish the body with protein, allowing you to lose weight throughout the day.

# HUMMUS Food of the desert people, eaten by millions in Africa, India, and the Middle East.

A Total protein will rebuild your immune system for cancer.

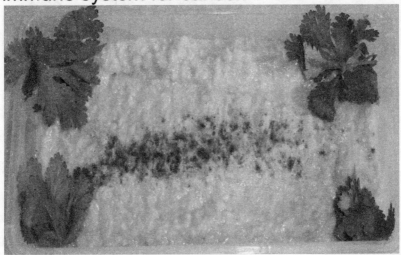

# TABOULI

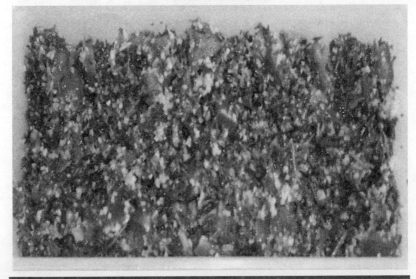

# TABOULI

**1.** Put one full cup of oats in a bowl of water even height to oats; let set until oats swell.

**2.** Get 2 bunches of parsley, pull leaves off stems, chop up real fine, put into bowl - don't put in stems.

**3.** Chop up 5 tomatoes real small, put into bowl.

**4.** Add one big onion chopped up into real small pieces.

**5.** Squeeze 5 lemons, take out seeds.

**6.** Add 1 ounce of GRAPE SEED OIL

**7.** When oats are soft enough to chew, they are ready to mix into the salad.

Stir and let set for about 2 hours – the longer it sets the better Tabouli is.

Tabouli is a good side dish to eat next to Hummus or to eat together on a 4 x 4 inch piece of pita bread, mustard green leaf, or lettuce, with a splash of lemon.

# MIDDLE-EASTERN PITA POCKET

**1.** Get pita pocket bread cut in half – shape of a half moon

**2.** Carefully open and spread a layer of lebni inside

**3.** Now spread layer of Hummus from Hummus recipe

**4.** Layer of Tabouli from my Tabouli recipe

**5.** Layer of sliced boiled egg

**6.** Three pieces of turnip pickles

YUM, YUM, YUM

# THE NO MEAT SANDWICH

**1.** Take pita bread, spread a thick layer of Lebni, hummus and/or tabouli inside. ADD mustard leaf , mushrooms sautéed in GRAPE SEED OIL, garlic, onion, tomatoes, etc.

Be careful not to chew on your tongue!

# VEGETABLE PITA POCKET

**1.** Get pita pocket bread.

**2.** One layer of lebni inside.

**3.** Chop cauliflower, broccoli, carrots, mushroom into small pieces, steam in covered pot for 15 min.

**4.** Place 3 spoons of vegetables in pocket bread and eat.

# RICE SALAD THE PARTY HEARTY

**1.** Cook 1 pound brown rice & drain rice, put in large bowl

**2. ADD** 1 cup pineapple,
  ½ cup green olives
  ½ cup raisins,
  1 cup chopped apple
  ½ cup tangerine,
  1 cup sliced banana
  1 cup green grapes cut in half

**3.** Add 1 pint of lebni, cottage cheese or yogurt

**4.** Cut 16 ounces of Colby cheese in to small pieces and put into salad stir up in large bowl with 1 cup small round tomatoes

**5.** Get a can of sliced beets lay to sliced beets on a plate, and place a line with 4 spoons of rice salad over the beets, and eat.

# HEALTHY TACOS

**1.** Get 1 high fiber whole wheat taco tortillas and Spread lebni, HUMMUS & salsa on tortilla

**2.** Add 2 spoons of tofu, chicken or lean ground turkey that has been fried in GRAPE SEED OIL with basil and chives.

# TOMATO CUCUMBER SALAD

1. Cut 3 large tomatoes into large pieces. Peel 3 cucumbers. Slice cucumber every 1/4 inch. Place in bowl with tomatoes
2. Now pour in ½ cup GRAPE SEED OIL and ½ cup of brown APPLE CIDER VINEGAR
3. 3 shakes of parsley, chives, basil, curry
4. Add 1 cup of cooked pasta to bowl.
5. Add 5 black olives and stir - mix in bowl.
6. Add goat cheese or any cheese you like.

# HOMEMADE PICKLES
# PICKELED CUCUMBER
## "The Sophia Snack"

1. Peel and slice 2 cucumbers, place in sandwich zip lock bag.
Add 2 shakes parsley, basil, curry, rosemary, cilantro, pinch of sea salt
Seal bag, shake bag a little.
Set bag in bowl in icebox - let set for one hour.
2. Take cucumbers out of bag, squirt lemon juice over the top, and eat. If you like, add a pinch of paprika over the top.

# PEANUT SAUCE "NUTTY BUDDY"

1. Put 5 spoons creamy peanut butter in pot
2. Put in 7 spoons of honey or 100% maple syrup,
3. Add 3 spoons of mustard,
4. Add ¼ once of GRAPE SEED OIL,
5. Squeeze the juice from one lemon,
6. Add 3 spoons of crushed peanuts, almonds, walnuts or pecans – whichever you choose.
7. Add 2 shakes of chive seasoning,
8. Add 1 shake of curry and sea salt,
9. Heat on low; warm - do not burn.

When all is melted, serve and enjoy.

# GARLIC PASTA IN BASIL SAUCE

1. Chop up 3 garlic cloves, put in pot of boiling water with ½ bag of pasta and 3 shakes of chives, boil 20 min.
2. Now put 1/4 cup of sour cream or lebni, 1 cup of GRAPE SEED OIL into a separate pot.
3. Add ½ cup of chopped tiny basil, 1 crushed garlic clove, pinch of sea salt, 3 shakes of parsley.
4. Cut 1 lemon in half, squeeze juice into basil sauce, and heat for 15 min on low.

# HEALTHY AMERICAN FRIES

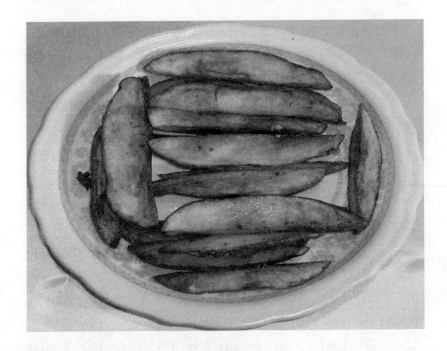

This recipe is pretty simple.
1. Wash off brown potatoes
2. Cut the potatoes the shape you like, horizontal or vertical
3. Place potatoes in pot, fill pot with GRAPE SEED OIL one inch from the top of the potatoes
4. Cook on medium high for 20 to 30 min.
5. After done, add sea salt
6. For kids, add 4 slices of cheese

Kids love these totally healthy fries.

# HEALTHY CASSEROLE

**1.** Spray the bottom of a Large Pot with GRAPE SEED OIL, put in 1 lb of mixed vegetables, & 1 lb of Tofu or Tuna

**2.** Add 2 cans of cream of mushroom soup.

**3.** Now 4 shakes of basil, curry parsley.

**4.** Chop two large onions and 3 garlic cloves - chop into pieces.

**5.** Cook a separate pot of 1 lb pasta. Rinse pasta.

**6.** Put everything into 1 pot, stir, and heat in the oven for 1 hr, 20 min.

**7.** Let cool down for 15 min, then put parsley trim around the circular or square pot.

# PIZZA BURGER

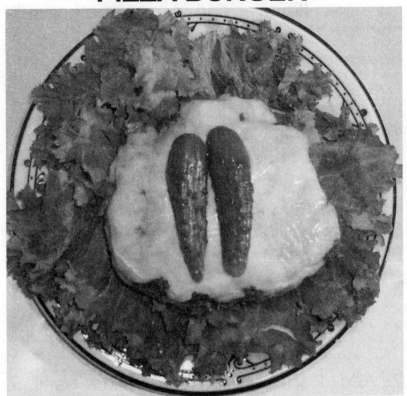

1. Spray GRAPE SEED OIL in frying pan; have ground tofu, turkey or chicken available.
2. Chop up parsley and mushrooms into tiny pieces - about 2 tablespoons of each.
3. Add 2 shakes of curry and sea salt to ground turkey
4. Mix parsley and chopped mushrooms into turkey patty

5. Fry medium low for 15 min on one side, then flip over and fry on the other side for 15 min.
6. When burger is just about ready, open small can of pizza sauce or tomato sauce and pour over burger
7. Now place one slice of mozzarella or Swiss cheese, put 2 slices of sweet or dill pickles on top of cheese, place lid over the pizza burger
8. Leave the lid on until cheese melts
9. Place on high fiber brown bun and enjoy.

# SWEET CORN

1. Get frying pan, spray 12 squirts grape seed oil, 1 spoon mustard.
2. Add 4 shakes curry, 4 shakes basil, 2 shakes parsley.
3. Add 7 spoons of maple syrup.
4. Cut 1 green onion into pieces.
5. Now 1 can of corn or fresh corn off cob. Cut 1½ cups.
6. Pour 2 ounces palmettos on top of corn.
7. Cook slow and low 20 min.
8. Place in bowl.
9. Don't forget to drink the juice when finished.

# VEGETABLE DINNER

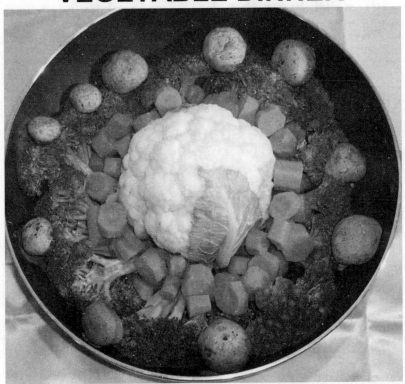

**1.** Get a large round pot. Place 1 large cauliflower in the center of the pot.

**2.** Now get 2 lbs of broccoli. Cut the stems of the broccoli long-ways through the broccoli so that the broccoli stems can lay under the cauliflower in the pot.

**3.** Now put mushrooms, one layer, ring around the cauliflower in from broccoli.

**4.** Put 1 layer of baby carrots in a ring closest to the cauliflower laying flat, going in a circle around cauliflower

**5.** Cook on slow and low for 30 min with a lid over the pot, preferably a round dome shape lid or another round shaped pot to cover while steaming.

**6.** After 25 min put a layer, maybe 5 slices, of cheese on and around the cauliflower dome shape and eat.

# LENTILS AND BLACK BEANS

**1.** Place 1 cup of lentils and 1 cup of black beans in a bowl

**2.** Add ¼ cup of brown APPLE CIDER VINEGAR, ¼ cup of Grape Seed Oil, add the rest water to make even with the top of the beans.

**3.** Let set till beans have soaked up the oil and the vinegar.

**4.** Take a spoon and take the foam off the top of the beans - we have just released 50% of the gas in the beans

**5.** Now place the beans in a pot, add 3 shakes of basil, parsley, rosemary, chives and curry, 5 spoons maple syrup.

**6.** Cook on low 2 hours until beans are soft to eat.

# MASHED POTATOES

1. Get large pot - spray inside the pot with GRAPE SEED OIL
2. Take 6 brown potatoes, wash them off real good
3. Now chop the potatoes up into medium chunks and put in the large pot
4. Add 3 cups of water, 1 cup of plain soy milk, turn stove to medium heat
5. Cook for 45 min, then add 8 oz. of mozzarella cheese - always keep stirring during your cooking process
6. 5 squirts of Grape Seed Oil
7. 5 shakes of basil, 10 shakes of chives
8. 1 tablespoon of sea salt
9. If you need to thicken, add 1 potato
10. Let cool down for ten min.
11. If you want gravy, cut up 3 onions, fry in skillet with 1 ounce of extra virgin olive oil till brown, add 3 spoons of wheat flour, a half-cup of water, and stir.

# HEALTHY ROLL UPS

1. Spray bottom of pan heavily with GRAPE SEED OIL
2. Add ¼ ounce of maple syrup or molasses and ¼ ounce of teriyaki sauce, on low in pan
3. Have 1 pound tofu, turkey or chicken ready
4. Now 3 shakes of basil, parsley, rosemary, curry, and a pinch of sea salt on turkey
5. Chop up 2 long stems of green onion
6. Chop up ¼ cup of parsley
7. Put all ingredients into turkey, roll turkey into little balls about half the size of a golf ball
8. Cook slow and low for 30 min.
9. Place toothpicks in turkey roll-ups
10. Serve on platter

# PARTY PÂTÉ

**1.** MIX a can of ground sardines.*

**2.** Add 3 Tablespoons honey or maple syrup

**3.** Add 2 large spoon of yellow mustard

**4.** Add 4 squirts of Grape Seed Oil

**5.** Add 2 shakes of chives and curry

**6.** Cut and squeeze the juice from one half of a lemon

**7.** Stir everything together

**8.** Taste and re-season if necessary. Pile into a shallow bowl and chill. Serve with high fiber chips or bread.


*Sardines substitutes = 1 pound of ground tofu, seafood, poultry, meat, vegetables **or** 4 eggs or 4 avocados

# TOMATO SOUP
## "BEAT THE BIG C"

1. Put 12 tomatoes in a pot.
2. 1 cup of GRAPE SEED OIL
3. ½ bunch of chopped basil
    ½ bunch of cilantro
    ½ bunch of parsley
    ½ bunch chives
    ½ bunch of green onions
4. 7 cloves of garlic cut in half
5. 4 shakes of original
6. 1/8 cup brown brown APPLE CIDER VINEGAR
7. 3 cups of distilled water
8. Cook on low for 2½ hours, stir for 2 min every half hour
9. One hour before done, add 2-ounce jar of palmettos and saw palmettos
10. Now add 3 tablespoons of maple syrup and stir.

# DRINK THE JUICE

# SUCCOTASH JUICE

1. Get one bunch of mustard greens, collard greens, turnip greens, spinach, and cabbage.
Chop up all green veggies about every 2 inches.
2. Fill the pot with water half the height of the greens in the pot. Add 10 squirts of GRAPE SEED OIL.
3. Shake 5 shakes of basil, chives curry, Cajun spice and paprika.
4. Chop 1 onion and 1 bunch of green onions real small.
5. Add ½ once of honey, 5 squirts of brown APPLE CIDER VINEGAR
6. Add 1 lemon cut in many pieces – add all parts of lemon and 5 cut-up garlic cloves into pot.
7. Stir all this up, cook on low for 4 hours, eat, and drink the juice. There is no pill that can compare with this juice.

# LEMON DRINK *VARIATIONS:*

**1.** Cut 8 to 10 lemons, put in a pitcher of water.

Let set four 4 hours.

**2.** Cut 8-10 lemons, put in picture of water.

Add warm ½ ounce of honey - be careful not to burn or overheat.

**3.** Same as #2 - this time add 5 pellets of bee pollen.

**4.** If sick with colds or flu,

Cut 3 lemons in half, Squeeze into a small pot, Take out the lemon insides, Drop into pot,

3 table spoons of honey,

3 table spoons of brown APPLE CIDER VINEGAR,

(the brown only), Crush 3 cloves of garlic chopped up real fine,

Add 4 ounces of water and one chopped up large mustard green curly leaf.

Heat your healing tea for 10-12 minutes.

This lemon drink helps to prevent colds, fight bacteria, viruses, inflammation on chest, flu, cuts mucus, stomach indigestion and **CUTS THE FAT.**

# POMEGRANATE JUICE
# A FULL POWERED DRINK
# "KING POMEGRANATE"

*Try different variations:*

1.  Pomegranate juice - one 4-6 ounce glass.
2.  Pomegranate Juice with 5 pellets of bee pollen - stir for 30 seconds.
3.  1/3 pomegranate juice, 1/3 cranberry juice, 1/3 red wine. Add a splash of lemon and 1 thin slice of lemon on top.
4.  2/3 pomegranate Juice, 1/3 apple juice.

Pomegranate juice fights cancer, restores kidneys, pancreas, bladder, allowing urinary tract to flow. Restores memory loss and helps vision, rejuvenates the brain, cleans and purifies your colon, stops blood clots in legs, and fights all toxins entering the brain.
The Highest of Liquid Antioxidants.

# POMEGRANATE SMOOTHIE
**Especially for the BLOOD, cancer, bladder, kidneys, pancreas, memory loss**

**1.** Have blender and chopped ice or ice cubes ready.

**2.** Cut up entire pomegranate fruit: hull, skin, seeds and all chopped into small pieces and placed into the blender with the 'Smoothie' recipe above.

**3.** Chop up 1 apple, 1 banana, 4 strawberries, 1 kiwi, 4 spoons of pineapple chunks.

**4.** Add a cup full of ice, 1½ cup of plain soy milk, and blend and drink.

POMEGRANATE rejuvenates vision for your eyes, allows blood to flow freely to the brain, increasing wisdom and knowledge. Restores the bladder and your kidney. In short pomegranate rejuvenates and purifies your blood as if you took it all out, washed it and put it back.

What a Godly blood cleaner the antioxidants in pomegranate juice does works miracles.

# SMOOTHIE for the THROAT
## *Dissolves and prevents THROAT cancer and throat problems*

Put into blender:

1 Banana

1 Apple

½ cup Pineapple

¼ teaspoon bee pollen

3 Whole Mustard Green Leaves- stem and all

Then add Soy milk, aloe vera or coconut juice to fill up the blender Blend and ENJOY!

# ALL-IN-ONE MILKSHAKE
# Especially for the skin

**1.** Put 1 Banana In Blender, Chop 1 apple, put in. Add 4 tablespoons of pineapple chunks, 4 strawberries, 1 carrot chopped, 2 kiwis, 1 peach, 6 Tablespoons of honey.

**2.** Add ice and soy milk,

**3.** 1 spoon of wheat germ,

**4.** 5 pellets of bee pollen, And blend.

This is the ultimate all-in-one health food drink - great for breakfast or lunch; it makes a pretty face by restoring skin cells.

# TOMATO JUICE

**1. For cancer:**

2 glasses of tomato juice a day,

Add one table spoon of vinegar per glass, one shake of basil, one shake of curry seasoning and 3 Tablespoons GRAPE SEED OIL

If you have no heart problems add one shake of paprika spice, stir and drink.

**2.** For general health, drink one glass of tomato juice 3 times a week.

Prevents and fights cancer, very high in antioxidants, enriches your blood, stops bacteria growth and stops cancer from spreading

# GRAPE JUICE

Drink 4 ounces, 3 times a week to promote good health and build a strong immune system.

10 times more vitamin C than an orange, fights colds, infections and bacteria, detoxifies the colon, promotes a regular bowel movement, fights cancer, helps clear dead cancer cell bacteria through the bowel tract, and keeps cancer from coming back.

Try to buy 100% Grape Juice only. It is better if you can find the juice not from a concentrate - that would be best. Raw grape juice is hard to find.

# PLAIN SOY MILK

1. Drink 1 glass a day to keep a strong immune system.
2. Drink 2 glasses a day to promote health, and for cancer patients.
3. Soy milk is high in calcium and makes you live long! We need 1500 mg of calcium a day to have perfect health. Some countries' mountain water supplies carry as much as 1000 mg of calcium or more. Average age 90 to 123 years of age.

# CABBAGE JUICE
## FOR THE BRAIN

Put 1 cabbage into a pot,

Fill with water to top of cabbage,

Add 4 shakes of curry,

7 squirts of brown APPLE CIDER VINEGAR,

7 squirts of GRAPE SEED OIL 8 Tablespoons

A pinch of mustard seeds

Add 2 shakes of cayenne pepper or 2 drops of habanera sauce,

2 cloves of garlic.

Cook on low and slow for about 2½ hours.

Eat, and drink the juice.

This is a brain food that helps headaches, tumors, aneurisms, and cancer.

# CONTINENTAL BREAKFAST

1. Grapefruit and 1 apple or orange,
2. 1 bran muffin, croissant or wheat toast,
3. 1 glass of milk or orange juice.

# GOURMET EGGS

1. Spray frying pan with GRAPE SEED OIL.
2. Whip in bowl 5 eggs, then stir in 3 shakes of garlic, parsley, basil, chives, 1 chopped up green onion, 4 chopped up mushrooms, 1 chopped up tomato, 3 Tablespoons GRAPE SEED OIL and 1 pinch of mustard seeds
3. Stir well, now pour into frying pan, stir well for 1 min, cook until eggs look 95% done. Turn off stove. Move the eggs to a different stove iron that was not turned on and let set for 5 min and eat. The eggs will finish cooking while they set.

# BREAKFAST BURRITOS

1. Package of wheat flour tortillas
2. Cook 2 cups of black beans.
3. Fry 5 eggs.
4. Peel cilantro from the stems - 1 full cup
5. Fry 8 strips of lean turkey bacon till it is semi hard so that you can crush it up.
6. Take 1 pint of lebni and start to spread lebni over tortillas, then add 1 large spoon of black beans, 1 spoon of egg, 1 spoon of cilantro, 1 spoon drained turkey bacon, 1 Tablespoons GRAPE SEED OIL and 1 pinch of mustard seeds.
7. Now make sure everything is in the center of the tortilla long-ways, fold the left side of the tortilla 1/3 of the way over stuffing, now fold the bottom and the top and roll the rest over, and heat and eat.

Home Cooking Cures ~ EAT to Heal the BODY!

# RED SNAPPER NUGGETS

1. Buy 2-3 pounds of red snapper, have your local store take fins, scales, and head off and cut into 4-inch chunks. Check the color - red snapper fish must look the color red. If it looks brown then it is not the true red snapper. The fish you buy should smell fishy, not stinky
2. Put 4 Tablespoons of GRAPE SEED OIL in frying pan.
3. Crack 1 egg, put in bowl, break yolk, and stir for 1 minute.
4. Have a plastic baggie ready with 3 ounces of corn meal. Add 3 shakes of basil, chives, Cajun, and 1 pinch of mustard seeds
5. Now dip the nuggets in the egg, making sure that all nuggets are covered in the corn meal. Take them out, put in bag with yellow corn meal, shake until all fish is covered, fry for 10 min. each side.

# SALMON CROQUETTES
## CORN CROQUETTES,
## WHEAT FLOUR CROQUETTES
## AND PANCAKE CROQUETTES

1. Get 2 cans of salmon, place in a bowl crush the bone of the salmon with a spoon until they look no more like a bone and stir salmon.
2. Crack 1 egg place in a bowl and stir.
3. Chop up 1 long stem of green onion into small pieces, MIX together: onion, egg, 3 Tablespoons GRAPE SEED OIL, 1 pinch of mustard seeds and salmon into patty.
4. Now place on a plate: 1 cup of yellow corn meal, wheat flour or wheat pancake mix.
5. Lay the salmon patty on the corn meal or the pancake mix, put flour on both sides of patty and fry for ten min, flip over, fry until it looks golden brown.
6. Take out and eat

# SLAMMIN' KING SALMON

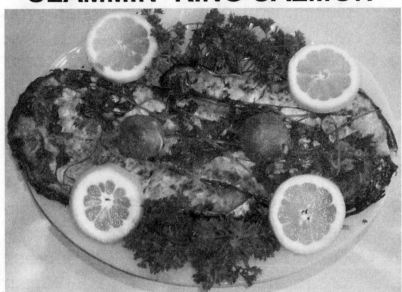

First, cover baking pan with a large sheet of aluminum foil, large enough to cover the fish and fold over the fish from both sides. Fold the sides together to seal so that no flavor gets out of the foil.

1. Spray the bottom foil in the baking pan with GRAPE SEED OIL.
2. Put a layer of parsley and cilantro mixed across the pan - do not cut off the stems.
3. Sprinkle basil, chives, Cajun, and curry seasoning in pan.

4. Cut 3 garlic cloves, chop into small pieces, and place in pan where you will put the fish.
5. Place salmon over the top of garlic, basil and parsley, curry and Cajun seasoning, spray top of fish lightly with GRAPE SEED OIL,
6. Put seasonings on the top the same as you did seasonings on bottom
7. Fold the foil together in the center, fold over and lock in flavor.
8. Cook in preheated oven at 325 degrees for 45 minutes, take out, let finish cooking while setting for 15 min.
9. Open foil, let set for 5 min, and eat.

# SHISH KABOB
# "JOLLIE KABOB"

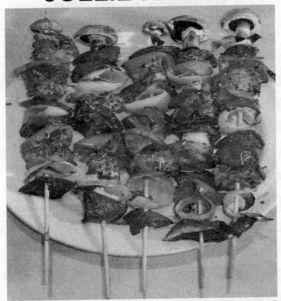

1. Get 4 pieces of breast of chicken or other chicken pieces. Make sure that all the skin is off, and wash the chicken – be careful of cross contamination in your cooking area. Cut 2-3-inch, small pieces.
2. Put chicken pieces, curry, lemon juice, basil, and spray 3 squirts or 3 Tablespoons of GRAPE SEED OIL, in a zip lock baggie, zip, and let set.
3. Get 3 green and 3 red bell peppers, 5 tomatoes,

4 brown onions. Cut up in 2-3 inch, small pieces.
4. Get one package of mushrooms, but do not cut the mushrooms.
5. Take the chicken out of the bag.
6. Get shish-ka-bob skewer sticks, slide onto stick, green bell peppers
7. 4 inches before the end of stick, now add a piece of onion, chicken, and tomato, red bell pepper, and onion.
8. Copy this sequence for all shish-ka-bob sticks. Place in a baking pan and cover.
9. Cook for 35 min - squirt with lemon.
10. Pour on BBQ sauce, Teriyaki sauce, honey, maple syrup, or just leave plain.

# MY LEMON CHICKEN
*This dish is one that kids also love.*

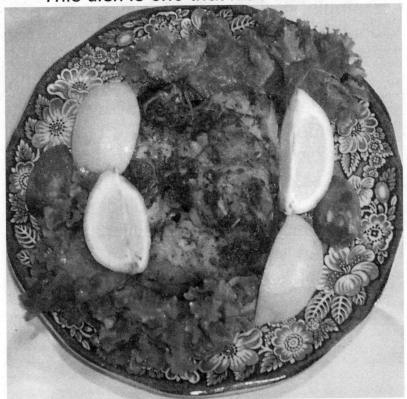

1. Put 4 Tablespoons GRAPE SEED OIL into a pan, plus five shakes of curry, parsley, basil, rosemary and a pinch of mustard seeds.
2. Put a layer of fresh cilantro and parsley in pan, remembering to leave the stems, do not cut.
3. Now put in 5 spoons of honey or 5 spoons of maple syrup,

4. For each piece/slice of chicken you plan to cook, cut and chop up one lemon. Example: 4 slices of chicken = 4 lemons; put the entire lemon in the pan including seed and lemon skin.

4. Put Chicken in pan, bottom side up, sprinkle fresh basil, parsley, and chives over the top.

5. Cook on low for 40 min, then flip chicken right side up, cook on low for 40 min. Lemon seeds and skin will dissolve into your sauce creating the Ultimate Lemon Chicken Meal

(Thin Chicken, cook 30 min, flip, cook 30 min.)

# FRIED CHICKEN

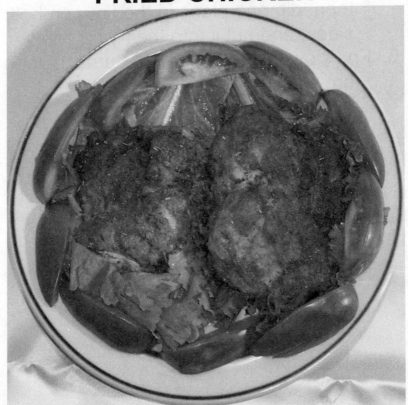

1. Put 8 Tablespoons GRAPE SEED OIL in skillet, and 5 shakes each of curry, basil, rosemary, garlic powder and 1 pinch of mustard seeds
2. Crack an egg, lay one large egg in a bowl,
3. Put one Cup of brown wheat flour on a plate

4. Soak the pieces of chicken in the egg then, dip one piece in the flour on both sides, and put it into the frying pan.
5. Fry slow and low until it turns golden brown.

# Mustard Green Chicken
## "The Green Chicken"

**1.** Spray pan with GRAPE SEED OIL

**2.** ADD 3 healthy shakes of curry, basil, parsley, chives, rosemary and garlic powder seasoning, 1 pinch mustard seeds, and 2 Tablespoons of honey.

**3.** Chop up 3 large leaves of mustard greens into 1½ inch pieces and spread across pan.

**4.** Put one layer of fresh cilantro and parsley mixed together. Spread across pan - do not cut the stems.

**5.** Now cut up two large tomatoes - spread them over the top.

**6.** Get 4-5 chicken breasts, place in pan bottom side up.

**7.** Now chop up 2 more large mustard leaves and spread over the top.

**8.** Last but not least, cut one lemon into 8 pieces and spread over top.

**9.** Cover with lid, cook on low for 35 min, then flip chicken over right side up and cook for 30 more minutes

**10.** Let cool down for ten minutes. Eat everything in the pan, don't forget to always drink the juice. Most of my cooking healing secrets are based on drinking the juice.

# TURKEY BURGER
## "THE JOLLIE BURGER"

1. Spray bottom of pan with Grape Seed Oil
2. Spread in pan, parsley and cilantro with stems
3. Chop 4 garlic cloves real tiny
4. Chop up ¼ bunch cilantro, ¼ bunch parsley without stems
5. Use 2 pounds ground turkey
6. Mix cilantro, garlic, parsley and 1 pinch of mustard seeds into turkey
7. Make a burger patty, now lay it over cilantro in pan
8. Fry on medium high for 15 min, flip and fry for 15min.
9. Add mozzarella cheese on top
10. Turn off stove, leave lid on top for 3 min.
11. Take off lid
12. Place burger on brown high fiber bread, never white, add one mustard leaf, one slice of tomato on top, and eat.

Bona Pâté!

# HOW I LEARNED TO COOK

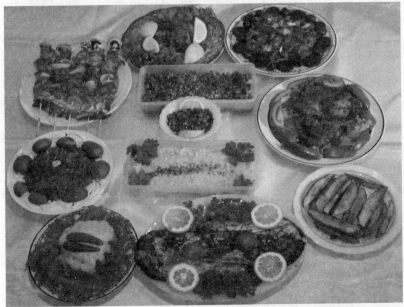

St. Louis Missouri - This is where my career began.

I use to wake up to the smell of my mother cooking early in the morning. I would be asleep, then that smell of home-made biscuits and eggs and sausage would flow past my nose, and I would jump out of bed and run down stairs to the kitchen. My mother was a very good cook. I use to watch her make different jellies and jams, peach cobblers and mincemeat pie. There were a lot of women in my family and they are all good cooks.

I love the smell of fresh apple butter. When I was 12 and in the Boy Scouts I baked a pineapple upside down cake. It was perfect, the best looking and tasting cake around. In my neighborhood it was all about whose mom could bake the best cake. There were many cooking pros within a few blocks. I showed my cake to several women in the neighborhood. No one believed I'd baked a cake on my own, they thought I'd bought it. Right then a light came on and a bell rang in my head. I knew I could cook.

From that moment on, I began baking blueberry, cherry cheese pies, etc., etc. And I haven't stopped.

I attended Northwest High School. In my freshman year I joined the varsity track team. The team excelled and managed to take state championship four years in a row. My specialty was the one and two mile relay. I was fast on my feet and ate a lot of food. I was eating so much my mother would scream, "You're eating me out of house and home."

In school I entered a "best dressed" competition where I came in second to a guy who called himself "pretty boy". Also during high school I worked at Lombardo's Italian Restaurant as a dishwasher to buy my clothes, have clothes tailor-made, and for free food while getting paid on the job. Pretty boy Craig's mother was sewing his clothes a mile a minute, and I was washing dishes at a mile a minute to get more money.

At the restaurant the cook's name was Andre - he was a French chef who went to school at Le Cordon Bleu in Paris, which was known to be the best culinary school in the world. Andre would do the old style cooking from 40 years ago. All types of fancy tricks while cooking; rolling lemons and oranges down one arm, across his back, and down the other arm. Andre would chop them up at the end like lightning. He was an amazing guy to watch. His cooking totally gave me goose bumps. I would go home with my mind simply blown just watching him cook one meal.

Sometimes Andre would take a cigarette break just to get out of the hot kitchen in the summer. He'd called me "Johnny Boy", and so did the owners,

Carmen, Gust and Angelo Lombardo. These guys were like my family and were also great people to work for. I had too much fun working for them during high school. One of my closest friends from high school named Ronald K. Pipes worked alongside of me. Those were some of the best days of my life.

Andre taught me to cook, so that when he went on a break, the kitchen would go on as normal. That way the orders would not slow down nor the kitchen gets backed up. Everyone in the kitchen was interchangeable if necessary. The ladies on the salad stations would come out and cook on the grill, in the oven, or go to the pizza station. Here I learned how to make veal scaloppini, frog legs, pizza burgers, and lasagna, rigatoni, fettuccini and eggplant parmesan, manicotti, linguine with clam sauce. The baked Alaska was my favorite, and the top of the line. We baked small ones and tall ones. One in specific was a light, tower shaped cake with a real light that came on inside the top of the cake. Baked Alaska's are cakes with the ice cream on the inside.

Later in life God blessed me with a job as a high-profiled personal assistant and high-profiled chauffeur to many royal families around the world. I have coached others, who have also traveled with royal families, on the protocol of being high-profiled chauffeurs and personal assistants for royal families.

While traveling throughout foreign counties, I've experienced the best foods for your body while eating in the finest restaurants. I've also had the opportunity of watching their cooks in action, while I picked up on old recipes. This is a blessing from God that has also helped me to calculate how to put these foods into a global order and pass them on to you.

My prayer is that this message will reach the homeless people for whom I will supply free food. This is also why I include international food stores as a part of my shopping. The mixing of the world's food is all part of the master plan that God has revealed to me. Cooking for cancer and AIDS patients is God's mission for me in life, and is my new goal.

# GOD'S FOOD
# CURES MANY DISEASES

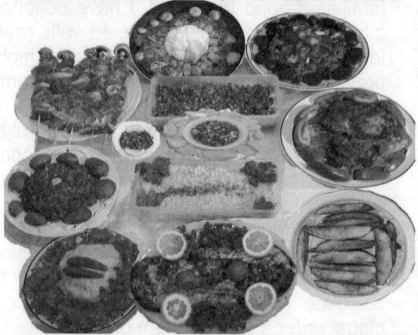

**CURES DISEASES Helping Senior Citizens** ★★★★★★★ I'm 78 lady. doctor had no answers for my sugar diabetes and failing kidneys.    Doctor sent me home to die..said that he could not help anymore.   ..since I have started this food program And praying to God     ..Now my doctor says that my kidneys and sugar diabetes are fine...thank you Jollie Harris for writing this book.    **Mrs. Hellen**

**An Inspiration** ★★★★★★★ ... advice on healthy eating .. has been tested and scientifically validated by medical & scientific institutions around the world. Great for Vegans and nonvegetarians. simple wisdom ... how to heal from your head to your toe. **Cancer Survivor Luther**

**SAVES YOU  MONEY & TIME!     NO DIETING,** Eat more, lose weight, regain health, vitality & stamina. Food secrets to restore & maintain your youth.    **NOW YOU,**  your family,  friends &  employees have THE SECRET to enjoy life, safely cure illnesses, prevent PAIN, surgery, and long hospital encounters.

# www.HomeCookingToCureCancer.com

## VIDEOS.HomeCookingCures.com
ISBN 1-4116-1065-2

53995

## AUDIOS.HomeCookingCures.com

9 781411 610651

# HOME COOKING TO CURE CANCER SONG

I drop down on my knees
To say a prayer
I need someone to talk to
But no one cares
I know that I'm lonely
Know that I'm in need
I want to say a prayer
to comfort me.
(Chorus 1)
Home cooking to cure cancer
And get your health back, too
Home cooking to cure cancer
Just might be the thing for you
(repeat chorus 1)
Some people live with
A lot of stress and pills
Oh, but they don't like
The way they feel
But when you got a problem
Remember God's food
Will solve them
He'll always make a way
You just keep the faith
(2nd Chorus)
You just keep the faith (4 times)
Now if you wake up one day
And the doctor say go away
Now if you wake up one day

So tired you can't stay awake
Remember keeping the faith
will bring you a brighter day
Home cooking the answer
To curing your cancer
Home cooking to cure cancer
And get your health back to
Home cooking to cure your cancer
Just might be the answer for you
Home cooking for cancer
And get your health back too
Home cooking for cancer
Just might be the thing for you
If you wake up one day
And your doctor says
Go away
Now if you wake up one day
So tired you can't even stay awake
Remember keeping the faith
Will bring you a brighter day
Home cooking the answer
I drop down on my knees
to say a prayer
I need someone to talk to
But no one cares
I know that I'm lonely
Know that I'm in need
I just want to say a prayer
To comfort me
( Repeat Chorus 1)  2X - 2 times
( Repeat Chorus 2)  4x - 4 times

# *TESTIMONIALS*

**Food that shrinks tumor in canine** [★ ★ ★ ★ ★] <u>bosco169</u>

About 6 weeks ago, I discovered a grapefruit size, protruding tumor under the stomach of our 13 year old golden retriever. Upon examination by the vet it was determined that he needed to have surgery to remove the tumor as soon as possible. The date was set for the following week. He proceeded to get so sick that we felt he might not live through the night. We took him back to the vet and it was determined that he had a bad infection and was given an antibiotic, which we did do. After speaking with the author of this book, HCTCC, we decided to postpone the surgery and try a natural alternative. I started feeding him the recommended foods from this book. I fed this to him daily for 2 weeks. His tumor began to shrink right away and about one month later, it is down to the size of a golf ball! His over health has improved tremendously. He can get up and down now, can bark again and has life in him again. I am so happy I read this book and I now use the food recommendations for myself and my family too!

**This Book is a must for everyone to read** [★ ★ ★ ★ ★] <u>Joan</u>

I was recently diagnosed with a mass on my ovaries and the doctor suggested surgery to remove the entire ovaries due to this irregular caused by this mass. I decided to go home and look into this matter. I went home and researched on what their surgery procedures would involve. Upon finding out I would possibly have to have chemo-and radiation treatments along with hormonal treatments, and doctor prescribed medications, I decided to look into holistic therapy.

Then, I also remember I had purchased Jollie's book in late December of 2004. I remembered reading of his idea in the book to help stop the cancer from spreading, while building the white and red blood cells and building up my immune system. I began trying this method for several weeks.

It has been a month and the bleeding has ceased since I adopted his method. I also eat the mustard greens raw and cook them as well. I also drink Pomegranate Juice to help build up armies of white and red blood cells to fight this disease.

I have not been back to the doctors office for a follow up and don't intend to. I am going to fight this disease using God's food! I made Red Bean soup and had cooked mustard greens on the side with rice. I have thrown out all white sugar and don't even drink milk unless it is soy or rice milk. Jollie, .. thank you for your wonderful book. I am very glad I bought it and it should be in every doctors office and part of their practice but sadly to say most people and doctors don't follow

God's way of healing. Bless you, my friend for your wisdom and effort into getting this information out to the public.

**THE HEALTH BIBLE** ★ ★ ★ ★ ★ ★  2 May 2007  by <u>Perry M</u>
JOLLIE THANK YOU FOR HELPING ME AND SO MANY OTHERS WITH GOD'S NATURAL WAYS TO HEAL THE BODY,KEEP UP THE GOOD WORK WITH YOUR MINISTRY YOU ARE GOD'S AMBASSADOR TO HEALTH. THIS IS THE BEST BOOK I HAVE EVER READ. MANY PEOPLE DO NOT KNOW GOD AND HOW GOD PUT FOOD ON THE EARTH TO HEAL THE BODY, OPRAH'S DOCTOR AGREES ON MANY OF THE SAME SUBJECTS THAT THIS BOOK IS TALKING ABOUT, MANY OTHER PEOPLE WHO BELIEVE IN NATURAL CURES FEEL THE SAME, SO THAT MEANS THAT HOME COOKING TO CURE CANCER IS THE BOOK TO READ TO HEAL ALL PARTS OF THE BODY. GOD BLESS THIS BOOK AND SHAME ON ANYONE WHO IS NOT IN AGREEMENT. RIGHT BEFORE PEOPLE DIE THEY WILL THINK ABOUT THERE HEALTH AND HOW THEY LEFT OUT GOD'S FOOD AS PART OF THERE DAILY PROGRAM.

**Leroy Jackson** ★ ★ ★ ★ ★ ★  4 Dec 2006 by <u>Leroy Jackson</u>
Hi My name is Leroy I am An Author & Poet who would like to say that this book is a 100% percent the true Native Indian way of healing the body through the Spirit of God. I know my grandparents are Native Indians. **This Amazing Book will be The Key To Your Health!** It's about time a book is released to the public that gets straight to the bottom line in a Godly way. I have read this book many times and got great results. .. Jollie in a simply way, eases the minds of everyone and tell the story of how God want us to heal the body in a way that a 2nd or 3rd grader could understand. Everyone should buy and have this book to secure their families.

**Simple Inexpensive ways to get healthy** ★ ★ ★ ★ ★ ★  <u>Luther</u>
I am writing this to let people know that this is the only book I could find that will give you the simple wisdom which God Has Gave Mr. Jollie Harris to express his Godly way of how to heal from your head to your toe. A great book for Vegans and nonvegitarians. The author of this book who is a messenger from God, is for sure doing God's Work. God said Knowledge is the Key and thanks for all the knowledge you have shared with me. Call Oprah Quick! God Bless the Author. **I AM A SURVIVING CANCER PATIENT** Believe me I have been surviving cancer for years now this is the greatest book you'll ever read it has helped me in so many different ways beat cancer. I have gave this book to my friend with aids and other sicknesses. This book works to heal any condition you may have now or have in the future. Buyer's buy this book and please disregard any

negative comments you may read buy others whom may try to write bad reviews about this book. I noticed that someone wrote a bad review This book and the Author are a blessing from God.

**Seriously Fab!** ★ ★ ★ ★ ★ 23 Oct 2006 by susjuly
You really have helped alot of people with this book I hope there is a part 2. It's brilliant that you can do that.

**Cured my Acid Reflex, NO more pills** ★ ★ ★ ★ ★ by Carla
This man changed my perspective on life when he cured my acid reflux disease and taught me how to eat to be completely healthy and preserve my body.. He cares for people in the deepest way possible. He instantly became my brother. My doctors said … take pills for the rest of my life. After I tried Jollie's suggestions, I stopped .. pills and have never since had any of my symptoms come back, and I know they never will. I am feeling the results for myself. I've never felt or looked better in my life! .. I have continued to eat his recipes on a daily basis and I have recommended the book to many of my family and friends, and all that try have been pleasantly surprised at the simple yet powerful effectiveness of this holy message. It's amazing how sensitive my body and mind has become to "outside" the plan of Gods food and in turn Gods plan for my life. The simple message of this book and food helps me relate all life situations and what is of GOD. In that way I was also spiritually healed. This man is a living testimony of how God turns the worst situations into the best possible. With his life experience, knowledge, and faith which allows him to confidently conquer even the most deadly diseases, he is a Devine intervention on our suffering sickly world.

I suggest this book to anyone who wants a REAL definition of being COMPLETLY healthy from any point in life or health status through the power of YOUR CREATOR.

**An Inspiration** ★ ★ ★ ★ ★ Anne Rogers
Although Mr Harris does not claim any qualifications nor particular expertise in his advice on healthy eating many of his opinions have been tested and scientifically validated by medical and scientific institutions around the world. This book will prove to be an inspiration to those who take the time to read it. And even if you are not a religious person one cannot doubt the wisdom of eating good wholesome food from natures garden. Mr Harris is on a crusade to educate the people of the world on how to eat a more healthy diet and I am in complete agreement with his ideas as I am on that same crusade with my own book.  author of A Guide To Healthy Eating

**Call Oprah Quick** ★ ★ ★ ★ ★ ★ 1 Oct 2004 by Luther Holmes
Somebody call the Oprah Show Quick and let her know that this amazing book is here! Everyone should adopt this food program.

especially Cancer & Aid's patients, regardless if they are on chemo/radiation or not. I am a surviving cancer patient who is getting back to his daily regular life of doing things for myself and my home. This food program which I have adopted and my trust in God has led me through the storm. Even my doctor has agreed that I am one of his fastest & strongest turn around patients that he has ever seen in his office. It is a blessing that this book has guided my immune system to regain full strength, and rebuild my blood cells. My Dr. is amazed that my blood pressure, sugar, weight and everything else is perfect. My PSA Count went from over 100% down to .01% Everyone should buy this book I give it 100 thumbs up If I could.

I have done very well on this food program for the past year and a half. I had 2 different types of severe cancer lung cancer and prostate cancer. ... .. bodies cant take the enormous amount of chemo poisons and as a result they pass away.

**THUMBS UP!** ✮ ✮ ✮ ✮ ✮ 21 Oct 2004 by <u>David Washburn</u>
I don't see how to give the rating.. But I just wanted to add, my thumbs up for you Mr Harris..

**GRATEFULL!!** ✮ ✮ ✮ ✮ ✮
I have been using the recipes and I find that I have no problem with it. My body is loving the change. I'm not tired and sluggish, I don't need to take antacids anymore.. My bowels are working better than ever... I can go on and on. I'm a young 65 and feeling like I did at 35-40. SO people make your own choice based on how you feel.

**Amazing Results** ✮ ✮ ✮ ✮ ✮ <u>janice harrison</u>
I am thankful that god has sent someone to cure his people in a natural way. I pray that all of his people receive this blessing, I have been reading this book for two weeks and have gotten amazing results. Thank you .. for all your knowledge.

**Amazing book.** ✮ ✮ ✮ ✮ ✮ 19 Oct 2004 by <u>tinhorn</u>
Fascinating recipes. God has given us everything we need for proper sustenance, including messengers. May He bless your work, Jollie. tinhorn author,

**Helping With My Heart Condition** ✮ ✮ ✮ ✮ ✮ ✮ I recently underwent a triple bypass heart operation. This book has helped me tremendously with my diet. Not only is it nutritious food but deliciously tasty the way it is prepared. This book is definitely a life saver. by <u>Raymond Lewis</u>

**Food and makeup** ★ ★ ★ ★ ★ ★ <u>MS. Ericka</u>
Dear Jollie, My mother gave me this book tonight to read and told me to give you a rating. At the time I was not interested in changing my diet. But after reading your book, I know that I can very well run into big health problems down the road. You are right we are what we eat. I will know pay closer attention to what I eat and the makeup that I wear. Keeping in mind that 2 out of every 4 women get cancer. Thank you for this book it will serve many people well.

**Christian Health Book** ★ ★ ★ ★ ★ ★ by <u>Marie</u>
Everyone in my family has bought this book and loves this book. We will also take this book to show the pastor's at our home churches, including the women and men's prayer groups. God Bless you and this book it is the way to perfect health. The Jackson's will support you where ever you go.

**Great Book** ★ ★ ★ ★ ★ ★ 8 Oct 2004 by <u>Herman J</u>
I knew it would be a great book when you first let me look through it and it was. I agree with every one else 10 THUMBS UP. Put this book on 20/20 OR NIGHTLINE, a news show.

**Helping women** ★ ★ ★ ★ ★ ★ 8 Oct 2004 by <u>Perry M</u>
God Bless you on your journey with your ministries of helping others who have cancer and other diseases and female problems.     There are many women in my family who appreciate your concern regarding cancer and how you solve the problem with food and the all mighty God's help! We thank you. Keep on being a Doer of God's work!

**This is a really great book** ★ ★ ★ ★ ★ ★ <u>Albert</u>
.. it is a lot better than I expected. It is also the way I use to eat when I lived down south in the country. ..

**Food That Works** ★ ★ ★ ★ ★ ★ 8 Oct 2004
I believe in everything you say. I have tried your cooking style and it works for me and my family, have noticed many

improvements in our health. God Bless you and I also hope that you get to cook on the Oprah Show. If you need a Fan Club President pick me. .. God Bless you. by <u>Popeye Vivian</u>

**10 Thumbs Up** ★ ★ ★ ★ ★ 8 Oct 2004 by <u>David Jackson</u>
I take my hat off to you what a great job of teaching people the correct way to eat I can't wait till your next book. I will always be a fan of yours. God will bless you.

**Schools & Corporations should read this book** ★ ★ ★ ★ ★
.. With a book like this you don't need health insurance. Boy you are going to save this country a lot of money by keeping people in good health! <u>Leroy Jackson</u>

**God's Health What a great book** ★ ★ ★ ★ ★ 7 Oct 2004
This is a wonderful book. It has all the info on the foods I need to keep healthy. I have really bad asthma and low energy. I have been blessed with the info in this book and have learned how eating the mustard greens solve my asthma and energy problems. Thank you Jollie Harris. Futhermore I am going to call the Jay Leno Show and the Oprah show, the world needs to know about your book. I will be your Fan anytime, start a fan club. by <u>Leonard Brown</u>

**Home Cooking to Cure Cancer** ★ ★ ★ ★ ★
This is a incredible book, the information in here is priceless. Jollie Harris seems to be writing from experience. I have tried some of the recipes in the book and the effects are amazing. Just using natural food instead of bottled pills. You just feel better immediately.  I totally recommend this book to anyone who wants     to     get     healthy     or     stay     healthy. This gets 3 thumbs up with a snap. <u>Lisa Calaway</u>

**Incredible! Blessed! Outstanding! God sent!** <u>darryl bocage</u>
This book is God sent. It gets back to the roots of what God wanted us to eat all along. My dog deja was very sick. I started giving her the mustard greens and bee pollen. She is now so healthy. God really works through this book. I started taking the

greens raw every day and the strength that i get is amazing. God bless you Jollie , I cant wait till the next book. Praise God!!!!!!!!

**Much needed resource!** ✮ ✮ ✮ ✮ ✮ by <u>Paris Hunter</u>
10 THUMBS UP!!!! I've read through the book and have tried many of the recipes.. The writer has given us a much needed resource for eating good food and how to prepare it ourselves. .. I .. recommend your book to my friends.

**A Cook book that Cures** ✮ ✮ ✮ ✮ ✮ ✮
This book is so great. God sent. I have been cooking for over 40 years. Now that I cooking from the recipes in this book my food taste better than ever. I feel like I am eating at a 3-5 star gourmet restaurant every day now. It's a great feeling to know that my food is now working to secure my health. My family has used this book to also cure colds,flues, allergies, asthma, bladder, sugar, blood pressure and all female hormone problems. This book will be a success on any and all talk shows. Thank God for the vision of Jollie Harris and helping my family. <u>Gloria</u>

**Home Cooking to Cure Cancer** ✮ ✮ ✮ ✮ ✮ ✮
I have read this book and think this book is a fantastic book. I had a very bad problem with diarrhea and could not eat anything. One of the things I found out was to eat mustard greens. This helps me to eat without having diarrhea all the time. I give this book a AAA+ I recommend it to everybody. Thank you Jollie Harris by <u>Tom Cavaness</u>

**keeping good health** ✮ ✮ ✮ ✮ ✮ ✮ 30 Sep 2004 by <u>Sophia</u>
The first time I read this wonderful book, I felt like this was a really good book and more people need to buy it and read it. Right when I read the first chapter I felt like I knew the author. God really has a reason for this man because the food really works and I would really recommend Oprah reading it , in fact I would like Oprah to do a episode featuring Jollie Harris and about how wonderful the book is . It is the best book I have ever read and I just hope Jollie Harris does another book. If you are out there and are reading this review I really recommend you buy this book right away because when you do you will be

happy with your look , health , and mind, and you will really understand how God's food works, so what are you waiting for , I am going to purchase my third book for my family.

**SAVES MONEY & TIME**  ✫ ✫ ✫ ✫ ✫  Lanette Randolph
What an intriguing book! I could not put it down. An autobiography AND a cook book! We really are what we eat. God's natural remedies have always been there for us, if only we would choose to recognize and use them. Thank you Mr. Harris for telling America like it is. America better wise up quick, especially WE FEMALES! Great book!!! Much future success to you and God Bless You.
NOpillsNObills.com

**Home cooking to cure cancer**  ✫ ✫ ✫ ✫ ✫  20 Aug 2004
by I believe this is the best book that I have ever read. This book gives you remedies from God with incredible recipes that really work. No pills no drugs just God's goodness from the planet. This book is truly a gift from God. I cannot wait for Mr. Star's new book. Praise God!!!!! cynthiabocage
[ 2 responses ] ✫ ✫ ✫ ✫ ✫  janice harrison
I have been reading the book only two weeks and I have seen great and I mean great changes in my body I thank you and I know you will bless many of gods people thank so much. bernardh I also believe it is better to trust God and eat right alot of times we don't have enough time to stop at home a cook everyone is to busy but we must make time to take care of our body that God gave us anyway. This book is a good way to start a healthy way of life with not sickness, diseases or problems. I know God is a healer but I rather not get sick. God bless you on your book and thanks.... Channel 9 and channel 2 news anchor men and women have quoted this book but God's food and the works of the author who helps people heal with God's program, have not yet been mentioned.

**FREE RECORDED BROADCASTS & SEMINARS:**
**www.VIDEOS.HomeCookingCures.com**
**www.AUDIOS.HomeCookingCures.com**

# HOME COOKING TO CURE
## RESTORE, REBUILD, REJUVENATE
## EAT TO HEAL THE BODY

--This International How to Cook Book has the answers, described fully with recipes using Our Creator's miracle foods, to prevent, reverse, reduce or cure/destroy worldwide CANCERS and most diseases. A simple to understand and follow food program not a diet, that shows How To use Our Creator's foods to make delicious, simple to make meals that will reverse: Cancers, Heart Attacks, Strokes, Seizures, Aids, Diabetes, Prostate cancer, Breast cancer, Uncontrollable Stomachs, Asthma, Glaucoma, Aneurysms, Alzheimer, Colds, Flu, Kidneys, Allergies, Female Menstrual, Hormonal & Menopause Problems, the Bladder, Blood Pressure, Pancreas, Lupus, ADD, ADHD, Acid Reflux, the Colon, restores Blood Cells, and Lose Weight, NO dieting, 5-7 meals per day...and much, much, more.

Paypal or send donations to feed & provide books to the homeless and those in need
1-888-432-5368  1-888-HEAL FOUNDATION

e-mail acure4cancer@yahoo.com regarding Home Cooking To Cure Seminars for churches, senior citizen homes, health clubs, large/small companies, and corporations. The price of this book is much less than A doctor visit.  You, your family, friends, associates & employees will save the high cost of surgery and long visits to the hospital.

## www.HomeCookingToCURECancer.com
## Feed God's Sheep Ministries

# NOTES: